~ *Naturally* ~
SKINSATIONAL

Rejuvenating Skin Care Recipes

SUE DOLAN

ISBN: 1-4392-1538-3
ISBN-13: 9781439215388

Visit www.booksurge.com to order additional copies.

*The first ever collection of natural anti-aging
skin care recipes that effectively promote facial rejuvenation
while treating a wide range of aging skin concerns.*

~ *Welcome!* ~

Hi! I'd like to introduce myself...

My name is Sue and I am the instructor and researcher for The Skin Care e-Learning and Resource Center. The Skin Care e-Learning and Resource Center is a website dedicated to providing current education on anti-aging skin care while focusing on facial rejuvenation strategies, techniques, and treatment options. We'd love for you to pay us a visit! ☺ To learn more about anti-aging skin care visit www.skincareresourcecenter.com.

I'm so glad that you are interested in caring for your skin with natural organic treatments. It's really a skinsational pleasure to meet you.

I'd like to start off by answering a few of the questions that I most frequently receive from those of you with inquiring minds. I know it might seem a bit unusual to have the FAQ right off the bat but I am certain that providing the answers to just a few of your questions will probably satisfy most of your curiosity.

As a result of my aging skin care research I became very interested in herbal lore and a natural approach to caring for aging skin.

It isn't that surprising since many facial rejuvenation products and medicinal treatments have their roots in using natural ingredients. Now enough about me, let's answer some of your other questions so that you can get mixing up your first batch of a wonderfully relaxing and rejuvenating facial treatment.

Naturally Skinsational was created to be a simple and fun recipe book with a focus specifically on natural anti-aging skin care recipes. Don't worry; you aren't going to find any obscure ingredients in any of these recipes that will require travel to a remote corner of the earth in order to make a simple rejuvenating facial mask. A natural skin care regimen just doesn't, (and shouldn't), have to be that difficult.

All the natural skin care ingredients used in these recipes can be found in your own cupboards or at your local markets. However, if you do happen to live in a remote rural area you might find it easier to order a few of the ingredients such as natural shea butter or nori seaweed through an online merchant. There are several excellent resources which have reasonable prices on online.

And yes, yes and yes. The natural skin care recipe card collections will be available very soon. I promise! I have heard from many people that they just love the idea of having their skin care recipes on good old fashioned recipe cards.

Feel free to download the free sample recipe cards that you'll find by visiting the natural skin care recipe page on www.skincareresourcecenter.com while I finish up working on the collections.

It's really quick and easy to create your own natural facial treatments for younger, healthier looking skin. Now get out your mixing bowl and start enjoying your rejuvenating natural skin care treatments. You are going to look absolutely skinsational!

Naturally,

Sue

~ *Disclaimer* ~

The natural skin care recipes included in this book focus on the treatment of aging skin concerns. These rejuvenating skin care recipes all feature natural ingredients which have known properties that can effectively treat aging skin issues. If you have specific questions regarding your use of any of the ingredients in any of these recipes please consult with your physician.

*If you have an allergy to
any of the ingredients;
do not use it!*

If you experience a reaction to any of the ingredients stop using it and consult with your physician. The author disclaims any responsibility or liability in connection with the use of these natural skin care recipes.

~ Table of Contents ~

Sue Dolan

~ Saving Face ~
Naturally

Every year people spend nearly 50 billion dollars on cosmetic products. And every year thousands upon thousands of new skin care treatments are introduced to the marketplace. The most recent trend is the creation and marketing of skin care formulas that highlight the use of natural ingredients.

The skin care industry has been capitalizing on natural ingredients as a foundation for many rejuvenating natural skin products. Products range from exfoliators and scrubs to toners and moisturizers that claim to effectively treat a variety of conditions including aging skin.

Just take a look at all the so called "natural" skin care products that have exploded onto the shelves in department stores, health food stores and grocery markets. Clearly, the pendulum is now swinging back towards a modern approach to the herbal lore of ancient times in order to treat a variety of skin conditions.

Why is natural skin care becoming such a phenomenon? The reason is quite simple, naturally! The sophisticated and complex set of properties found in natural ingredients such as antioxidants, proteins, vitamins, enzymes, and other plant nutrients that are commonly referred to as phytochemicals simply are not as effective when duplicated synthetically.

Herbalists have always known that the chemical ingredients in herbs work together holistically to facilitate facial rejuvenation. The active properties of herbs can have a significant and powerful effect that cosmetic companies can only hope to duplicate.

Manufactured products containing natural ingredients also begin to lose their potency almost immediately despite claims to the contrary. That's because products need stabilizers and preservatives to maintain a reasonable shelf life.

The organic skin care treatments you prepare can be just as effective as those high-end department store products and they certainly represent a significant savings.

The art of natural skin care makes use of natural ingredients you can easily find right on the shelves of your own pantry and in your garden. The lost art of herbal lore is making a comeback and with good reason. It works!

Natural skin care products not only work just as well as products that are formulated by cosmetic companies in treating many aging skin care concerns, but they are also wonderfully fresh and ridiculously inexpensive. Best of all, making your own skin care treatments is really a whole lot of fun!

Imagine finally being certain exactly what is in your skin care treatments. You control the quality of the ingredients. You can also easily tailor any recipe to meet you own specific skin care needs.

The art of natural skin care embraces the use of fresh, quality ingredients in order to achieve maximum effects.

There is a wealth of natural skin care ingredients with properties that will specifically treat aging skin.

- Rosemary
- Sage
- Mint
- Licorice
- Fennel
- Lactic Acid (found in many dairy products)
- Rose petals
- Rose hips
- Fresh fruit
- Honey

Ancient civilizations used a variety of skin care treatments. One of the most notable was honey. The classical Greek beauties used honey as a moisturizer to keep their skin soft and youthful. Honey is also a natural antibacterial agent. People believed that Cleopatra regularly soaked in a rose petal and milk bath to keep her skin soft. The rejuvenating properties of rose petals and rose hips have long since been scientifically documented.

For centuries the European gentry used dairy products to soften the skin. Olive oil is still considered the secret skin rejuvenating ingredient for Italians.

An amazing range of herbs is still used medicinally around the world. Herbal lore continues to be passed down as it has been throughout the ages while new beneficial medicinal effects of plant properties continue to be discovered and studied.

* SKINSATIONAL TIP:

Compresses of Vitamin C when applied to skin ulcerations encourages healing that rivals that of modern day antibiotics.

Organic natural skin care recipes offer a fun way to experiment using common items found right in your own kitchen, the local market or your own garden. An amazing array of combinations provides aging skin with wonderfully refreshing facial treatments that will promote a youthful and healthy appearance.

Even ancient beauties knew the fundamentals of maximizing the use of natural skin care ingredients and proved that they were able to effectively treat an array of skin conditions; you too will soon master the art of rejuvenating your skin naturally.

Use fresh ingredients to get the maximum benefit from the rejuvenating properties inherent in each recipe. Take a few moments on your next shopping trip and treat yourself to a few fresh potted herbs plants. If you don't have any yard space to create a small garden, use a planter. If outside plantings aren't an option, try growing a few potted herbs on a sunny windowsill. Most herbs are very hearty and will tolerate most environments if given a little sun and occasional water.

Next, stock your pantry with your favorite natural skin care ingredients and you'll be all ready to start mixing together your own wonderful rejuvenating facial treatments at any time.

Start whipping up your own homemade skin care treatments and rediscover your youthful, baby soft skin all over again!

~ Skin Essentials ~

A major goal in formulating a natural anti-aging skin care regimen is to select effective combinations of natural skin care ingredients to incorporate into your overall regimen that will address your specific aging skin concerns.

In order to reverse the signs of aging skin an important cornerstone of facial rejuvenation is to stimulate skin cell repair by accomplishing the following very specific, yet critical criteria:

- ❀ *Encourage collagen production*
- ❀ *Increase the skin's moisture content*
- ❀ *Improve the skin's ability to protect itself*
- ❀ *Neutralize skin damaging free radicals*
- ❀ *Stimulate skin cell renewal and repair*

The skin's natural ability to keep itself looking youthful and healthy diminishes over time. Natural anti-aging skin treatments provide visibly deteriorating facial appearances with the resources needed to protect the skin from further damage as well as to encourage the repair and rejuvenation process.

* *

* SKINSATIONAL TIP:

Skin needs proper nourishment inside and out to stay healthy. A balanced diet, adequate exercise and sufficient sleep play a vital role in youthful looking skin.

* *

During the aging process, skin gradually undergoes visible changes in skin tone and complexion. With age, the body's metabolism slows down. As circulation becomes more sluggish, the skin gets short-changed on the nutrients it needs to stay youthful and vibrant.

As these changes occur facial skin begins to sag, becomes much drier and starts to lose its elasticity. Aging significantly slows down the skin's ability to heal itself. Even small abrasions and bruises take longer to heal while blemishes take longer and longer to go away.

Highly charged oxygen molecules called "free radicals" make a significant contribution to the deterioration of the skin's condition. They are almost exclusively responsible for the visible deterioration of the skin which is evidenced by fine lines, age spots, wrinkles, and a host of other aging skin conditions. The presence of free radicals typically occurs as the result of too much sun, environmental pollutants, a poor diet, smoking and stress. All these factors accelerate the skin's aging process.

Fortunately, free radicals can be neutralized by antioxidants which are found as a rather powerful property intrinsic to many of the natural skin care ingredients. But, (and this is a big but), in order to keep free radicals and their adverse effects contained, good facial skin care means using sunscreen on a daily basis; antioxidants just can't do it alone.

And, in case that's not enough, aging skin is also affected by changes caused by the gradual decrease in the production of elastin and collagen which adversely affect the skin's plumpness and suppleness. The skin's firmness deteriorates which contributes to sagging. The gradual loss of elasticity also promotes those dreaded wrinkles to deepen, initially beginning as fine lines that gradually turn into pronounced wrinkles as time progresses.

Bear in mind that stress, smoking, sun, insufficient sleep, excessive alcohol, lack of exercise, and poor diet all have a profoundly negative impact on the health of your skin. Some of the major characteristics that all these activities have in common are wrinkle acceleration. An unhealthy lifestyle provides an ideal environment for free radical activity which promotes sun damage giving birth to those brown spots as well as for the drying and sagging of skin to occur.

Add all these skin damaging factors together and a good corrective action plan is in order, a simple yet effective natural rejuvenating facial skin care treatment regimen.

A simple, basic, skin rejuvenation regimen increases the skin's moisture content, stimulates collagen production, neutralizes free radicals, locks in the skin's own natural moisture, stimulates repair, and encourages the skin's own natural defenses to work harder to protect itself.

The natural skin care ingredients needed to accomplish these goals are those which have the properties that will provide the skin with all the essential natural reinforcements necessary to address the visible signs of aging.

Fight the signs of aging skin with the following:

Antioxidants repair the skin and protect it from further damage caused by free radicals. Over time the skin builds up a reservoir of antioxidants that help to minimize sun damage by providing both protection and by stimulating cell repair.

Astringents cleanse the skin. They also help to draw tissues together causing proteins to coagulate, dry and then harden. This tightens skin tissues and reduces pore size, protecting the skin against environmental damage.

Demulcents calm inflamed skin and soothe irritated skin.

Emollients soften and soothe sensitive, dry skin.

Exfoliation encourages new skin cell growth by eliminating the outermost layer of older dead skin cells. Exfoliation can be accomplished in two ways. The mechanical exfoliation method uses a scrub. A chemical method uses a natural acid such as citrus juice. Exfoliation is one of the most basic and important steps in stimulating improvements for aging skin.

* SKINSATIONAL TIP:

Exfoliation renews skin by removing old skin cells and stimulating new skin cell growth.

Humectants help the skin retain moisture by actually holding moisture to the skin.

Moisturizing adds moisture to the skin by hydrating and locking in the skin's own natural moisture content.

Give your skin the resources it needs to protect itself from the myriad of aging skin symptoms.

All the ingredients included in the natural skin care recipes that you find in this book were selected for their rejuvenating properties and combined in simple formulas to effectively address a wide range of aging skin concerns.

Now take a quick peek at the natural skin care glossary to identify some ingredients that are suited for your skin type and aging skin concerns. The natural skin care ingredient glossary is short and sweet with only the essential properties described for each ingredient... honest!

---

* SKINSATIONAL TIP:

Sunscreen is a critical component of any aging skin care regimen. Antioxidants, exfoliants and moisturizers simply can't provide all the necessary protection the skin requires against the aging impact of sun damage.

~ Getting Started ~

First, quickly scan the glossary of natural skin care ingredients at the end of the book to identify which ones are best suited for your skin type.

Oily and acne-prone skin benefit most from ingredients with astringent and antibacterial properties such as rosemary, dandelion and plain aspirin. Normal skin types reap advantages from an array of combinations to maintain the skin's natural balance such as rose hips, fruit acids, and honey. Sensitive and dry skin types benefit from ingredients with emollient and moisturizing properties.

A quick synopsis of ingredient attributes best suited to skin types can be summarized as follows:

❀ *Oily Skin:* Astringents, antibacterial, antiseptic, antibiotic, anti-inflammatory, antimicrobial, antioxidant, cleansing detoxification, disinfectant, exfoliant, healing, cell repair

❀ *Normal Skin:* Antibacterial, antibiotic, anti-inflammatory, astringent, cleansing, demulcent, emollient, exfoliation, healing, hydration, moisturizing, cell regeneration, softening agent, stimulant

❀ Dry, Sensitive Skin: Antibiotic, cleansing, demulcent, emollient, exfoliation, healing, hydration, moisturizing, cell regeneration, softening agent, stimulant

As you will note, each skin type can benefit in some way from the attributes provided to the skin by natural ingredients. All ingredients and the properties they impart to the skin are interchangeable.

Balance your skin's needs with the properties of natural ingredients. For example, those with oily skin would prepare recipes that combined ingredients with astringent properties while those with sensitive skin would focus on recipes with ingredients that provided soothing and emollient properties.

By quickly reviewing the natural skin care glossary it will become easier to decide on the properties of the ingredients and those recipes that will best address your skin type and skin care issues.

Oily skin types will want to focus on ingredients such as citrus and exfoliating salt or sugar scrubs while sensitive skin types will want to include ingredients such as olive oil, dairy products and honey. Once you understand these basic principles you will soon be creating recipes that you have customized for your own skin's particular needs.

Begin by taking an inventory of the natural skin care ingredients available in your cupboards and refrigerator. The most common items include citrus fruits, dairy products, sugar, salt, vinegars, aspirin, eggs, honey, oatmeal, olive oil and tea bags.

Start slowly and add just a few new items to your grocery list each week. Making your own facial rejuvenation treatments should not be hard or overwhelming. It's really quite simple and fun. Not to mention how naturally skinsational it is to whip up a refreshing toner that not only cleanses but rebalances your skin.

All these recipes are quick and easy to prepare and invite your own creative touches. For the city dwellers, don't worry that you can't go outside to pick fresh dandelions. Just substitute another astringent instead. It's not a problem, honest!

Develop a natural skin care routine that incorporates cleansing, scrub, toning, and moisturizing recipes using the natural ingredients best suited for your skin type. For example, a person with normal skin might use a sea salt scrub recipe followed by a lemon juice toner and an olive oil based moisturizer.

* SKINSATIONAL TIP:

Don't be afraid to adapt any of the recipes or tailor the ingredients to suit your own particular skin care needs. There is absolutely nothing wrong with adding a bit of mashed banana to a recipe if you want to add a moisturizing element or adding a squeeze of fresh lemon juice to help bleach out those age spots.

It's helpful to collect a few small glass or plastic containers which will make it easy to store your homemade facial treatments.

You'll also need a small spray bottle for facial mists, a small bottle for toners, a funnel, and a small colander or strainer. All these items are readily available at most grocery stores, drugstores or large department stores. The travel size plastic bottles for toiletries work very well for storing leftover facial mixtures.

Its fun!
Let yourself enjoy and experiment so you can discover
which ingredients and recipes work
the best for you and your skin.

Most natural skin care recipes can be made ahead and will keep for several days when refrigerated. Many can even be frozen in individual treatment sizes so don't be afraid to pull out the big mixing bowl.

There are literally thousands of natural skin care recipes that will address a wide range of skin care issues from combating acne outbreaks to healing skin irritations. The more you experiment with recipes the greater the success you will have in establishing your own effective natural skin care regimen!

* SKINSATIONAL TIP:

Vitamins C and E are critically important in maintaining healthy skin by stimulating normal cell growth.

Now you're all ready to get started!
Start mixing up your own healthful and
rejuvenating skin care products.

~ Facial Scrubs ~

Skin care recipes for facial scrubs are a wonderful way to exfoliate and condition your skin for very little effort or expense.

Exfoliation is accomplished by either a mechanical means when using a scrub or a chemical means by using an alpha hydroxy acid (AHA) or beta hydroxy acid (BHA). Exfoliation helps to remove old, dead skin cells that collect on the surface of the skin as well as to encourage the growth of new cells while stimulating the production of the ever important collagen.

The skin benefits significantly from exfoliation by not only becoming softer and more subtle but exfoliation helps in diminishing fine lines and wrinkles, in firming sagging skin, and contributes to evening out a mottled skin tone.

Many of the rejuvenating skin care recipes include a mechanical exfoliant ingredient such as a mild abrasive like salt, sugar or plain aspirin (BHA) as well as a chemical exfoliant such as a fruit acid (AHA) in the form of freshly squeezed juice from a citrus fruit. The abrasive serves to gently dislodge dead skin cells in order to reveal the new, healthier cells underneath. Scrubs also help to deeply clean pores which is extremely beneficial in reducing acne outbreaks and the reoccurrence of blackheads.

Scrubs are most effective when used on warm, moist skin. Prior to using a scrub simply apply a warm face cloth to your skin for a few minutes then gently use a circular motion to massage the scrub lightly on the skin.

* SKINSATIONAL TIP:

If you are allergic to certain foods, herbs or plants don't use them in a natural skin care recipe!

~ Exfoliating Aspirin Facial Scrub ~

- 5 to 10 of plain aspirin- the cheap generic kind is just fine
- 1 to 2 teaspoons of your favorite fruit acid; freshly squeezing the juice from a lemon, lime, orange, or grapefruit

Crush aspirin tablets into a fine powder- a small coffee grinder works really well if you are making a large batch. Mix well with the citrus juice adding only a one teaspoon at a time to make a thick paste. Use scrub prior to cleansing and toning in the morning.

This recipe is extremely versatile and can easily be adapted to suit any skin type. For a refreshing and exfoliating aspirin toner use a least 1/3 cup of freshly squeezed fruit juice to make a thin solution that can easily saturate a cotton ball.

* SKINSATIONAL TIP:

*Aspirin is salicylic acid, a beta hydroxyl acid.
BHA is frequently used as an active ingredient
in skin care products for oily skin types to promote
exfoliation as well as to treat acne prone skin.*

~ Enchanted Primrose ~

- 1/4 cup primrose petals
- 1 tablespoon walnuts
- 2 tablespoons pineapple juice

Finely grind the walnuts then finely chop the primrose petals. (A mini food processor works well.) Freshly squeeze the juice from a few slices of pineapple and mix all ingredients together well.

Gently massage into skin. Rinse well with warm water.

* * *

~ Honey Almond Facial Scrub ~

- 1 tablespoon of honey
- 2 tablespoons almonds
- 1/2 orange
- 1 mint leaf

Grind almonds until finely ground in a small food processor or coffee grinder. Finely chop the mint leaf then freshly squeeze the juice from the orange. Add remaining ingredients and mix well.

Gently use to scrub your face. Rinse well with warm water.

Any unused portion may be kept for up to a week in the refrigerator.

* * *

~ Acne Allies Scrub ~

- 1 tablespoon Epsom salts
- 1 teaspoon sage leaves
- 2 teaspoons fresh thyme
- 1/8 cup ripe mango

Remove the herb leaves from the woody stems of the sage. Peel the skin then roughly chop the mango. Combine ingredients in a food processor and pulse together until all ingredients are finely chopped and the mixture begins to form a paste.

Use to gently scrub face. Rinse well with warm water.

* * *

~ Lavish Lavender Scrub ~

- 1/8 cup lavender petals
- 2 tablespoons dark brown sugar
- 2 tablespoons grapefruit juice

Finely chop lavender petals then freshly squeeze the juice from a generous slice of grapefruit. Mix together with the brown sugar and citrus juice until smooth.

Gently massage into skin. Rinse well with warm water.

* * *

~ Simple Cleansing Scrub ~

- 5 to 8 tablets of regular aspirin (plain generic brand)
- 1 teaspoon of vitamin water

Crush the plain aspirin tablets into a fine powder. (A mini food processor or coffee grinder works well.) Slowly add a few drops of the water at a time until a thin paste forms.

Gently use to scrub your face. Rinse well with warm water.

* SKINSATIONAL TIP:

Slightly dampen a plain aspirin tablet and rub it on blemishes as a quick spot treatment for acne. The salicylic acid in aspirin is a proven effective treatment for acne.

~ Conditioning Scrub ~

- 2 tablespoons of coarse sea salt
- 1 tablespoon of honey
- 2 to 3 drops of olive oil

Mix the salt and honey together well. Slowly add the olive oil a drop at a time and stir until well combined and a thick paste forms.

Use to gently scrub skin. Rinse well with warm water.

* * *

~ Skin Softening Scrub ~

- 2 tablespoons of cornmeal
- 2 to 3 teaspoons of buttermilk
- 1 teaspoon of coconut oil

Combine all ingredients and mix together will until a thick paste forms.

Use to gently scrub skin. Rinse well with warm water.

* SKINSATIONAL TIP:

For generations cornmeal has been mixed with fresh citrus juice or a dairy product and used as a quick and easy absorbent cleansing scrub.

~ Citrus Exfoliating Scrub ~

- 1 tablespoon of honey
- 1/4 cup granulated white sugar
- 1/2 lemon, lime or orange

Mix together the honey and sugar, combining well. Slowly drizzle in the freshly squeezed citrus juice mixing ingredients into a thick paste.

Use to gently scrub skin. Rinse well with warm water.

* SKINSATIONAL TIP:

Use a wedge of fresh citrus fruit such as grapefruit, orange, lemon or lime dipped in sugar or salt for a refreshingly quick and easy exfoliating facial scrub.

~ Moisturizing Scrub ~

- 1 tablespoon raw sugar
- 1 tablespoon plain yogurt or buttermilk
- 1/2 teaspoon honey
- 2 teaspoons cream of tartar

Combine all ingredients until thoroughly mixed and a thick paste forms.

Use to gently scrub skin. Rinse well with warm water.

~ Herbal Hydrating Scrub ~

- 1/4 cup brown sugar
- 1/8 cucumber
- 4 witch hazel leaves
- 2 teaspoons fresh sage
- Drizzle of extra virgin olive oil

Place all ingredients into a food processor and pulse just a few times. Slowly drizzle in enough olive oil while pulsing to form a smooth paste.

Use to gently scrub skin. Rinse well with warm water.

....

* SKINSATIONAL TIP:

Witch hazel is a wonderful home remedy for many types of skin inflammations, burns and swelling.

....

~ Vitamin C Exfoliating Scrub ~

- 2 tablespoon coarse sea salt
- 1/2 orange

Grate the rind from the half orange then squeeze the juice. Mix the juice with the sea salt.

Use to gently scrub skin. Rinse well with warm water.

~ Sugar and Spice Facial Scrub ~

- 1 tablespoon of sugar
- 1 tablespoon cornstarch
- 2 tablespoons of buttermilk
- 1/8 teaspoon each of cinnamon, nutmeg, and cloves

Freshly grind each of the spices and mix together thoroughly with the remaining ingredients.

Lightly massage scrub into facial skin. Rinse well with warm water.

* SKINSATIONAL TIP:

Make a big batch of your favorite scrub recipe and store it in an airtight container to use throughout the week. Note: Recipes using a dairy product will need to be stored in the refrigerator.

~ Cleansing Grains ~

- 1 tablespoon bran
- 1 1/2 tablespoons plain yogurt
- 1 tablespoon wheat germ

Mix all ingredients together into a stiff, smooth paste.

Gently massage into skin. Rinse well with warm water.

* * *

~ Herbal Scrub ~

- 1 teaspoon fresh oregano
- 2 teaspoons fresh parsley
- 1 teaspoon fresh marjoram
- 2 tablespoons freshly squeezed lime juice
- 1 tablespoon sea salt

In food processor pulse ingredients together until well mixed and the herbs are finely chopped.

Use to scrub skin gently. Rinse well with warm water.

* * *

~ The Naturalizer ~

- 1/2 passion fruit
- 1 inch piece ginger root
- 2 tablespoons wheat germ

In food processor pulse ingredients together until all ingredients are finely chopped and mixed well.

Use to scrub skin gently. Rinse well with warm water.

* * *

~ Cornmeal Scrub ~

- 1/4 cup cornmeal
- 1 tablespoon ginger root
- Dash of light cream
- 5 grapes

Finely grate the ginger root. Combine all ingredients in food processor and pulse together until well mixed.

Gently massage into skin. Rinse well with warm water.

---

* SKINSATIONAL TIP:

Tartaric acid, a natural form of alpha hydroxyl acid, is a very gentle exfoliant found in grapes, wine and cream of tartar.

~ Limeaide ~

- 1/8 cup rolled oats
- 1 lime
- 2 tablespoons honey

Finely grate the rind of the lime into a small bowl. Then squeeze out all the juice of the lime into the bowl and combine with remaining ingredients. Mix together well.

Gently massage into skin. Rinse well with warm water.

* * *

~ Cranberry Cleansing Scrub ~

- 1/4 cup fresh cranberries
- 1/2 lemon
- 2 tablespoons sugar "in the raw"

Roughly cut lemon, skin and all into chunks. Combine all ingredients in a food processor and pulse until finely chopped.

Use to gently scrub the skin. Rinse well with lukewarm water.

* * *

~ Purple Passion Scrub ~

- 1/2 passion fruit
- 4 to 5 purple grapes
- 1 tablespoon kosher salt
- Scant teaspoon of balsamic vinegar

Combine all ingredients together in a food processor. Pulse until mixture is smooth.

Gently massage into skin. Rinse well with warm water.

~ Brown Sugar Scrub ~

- 1/8 cup brown sugar
- 1 tablespoon honey
- 1 tablespoon plain yogurt

Combine all ingredients in a bowl and mix together well.

Gently massage into skin. Rinse well with warm water.

* * *

~ Winterizer ~

- 1 carrot
- 2 tablespoons of cream
- 1/8 teaspoon whole cloves
- 2 to 3 small witch hazel twigs
- 1 tablespoon sea salt

Finely grate carrot then grind both the cloves and witch hazel in a coffee grinder. Combine all ingredients into a blender and whip together until smooth.

Gently massage into skin. Rinse well with warm water.

~ Acne Revenge ~

- 3 dandelion leaves
- 1 dandelion flower
- 1 tablespoon baking soda
- 1 lime
- 6 crushed plain aspirin

Squeeze the juice from the lime then pulse all ingredients together in food processor until thick and creamy.

Gently massage into skin. Rinse well with warm water

* * *

~ An Aspirin A Day ~

- 1 tablespoon cider vinegar
- 8 plain aspirin

Finely crush the aspirin tablets or grind them in a coffee grinder. Add the cider vinegar and mix together well.

Gently massage into skin. Rinse well with warm water.

* SKINSATIONAL TIP:

*Aspirin, a form of salicylic acid, can be crushed
and formed into a paste to be used as a very effective
exfoliating treatment.*

~ Facial Masks ~

Facial masks (or masques) have been used since ancient times to soften and nourish the skin, unclog pores as well as to remove any impurities that remain after cleansing.

Homemade masks accomplish a variety of skin essential tasks by providing a means to convey critical nutrients to skin cells and deeply hydrate the skin by replacing the vital moisture content that so often fluctuates in aging skin. Masks also provide an opportunity for exfoliation as well as to condition and moisturize the skin.

Natural skin care ingredients that have emollient, antioxidant, and demulcent properties are traditionally incorporated into facial mask treatments along with those ingredients that hydrate and exfoliate. Homemade facial mask recipes are an especially effective strategy for rejuvenating aging skin. It goes without saying that they provide a wonderfully luxurious and relaxing experience.

Facial Masks are used to draw a fresh supply of blood to the skin in addition to replacing lost moisture, and stimulating circulation to the facial area. The nutrients in natural mask recipes help to stimulate cell renewal, tone and firm the skin. Masks are also an excellent way to give your skin a deep pore cleansing to facilitate healing and overall skin health.

It's time to get out your whisk and mixing bowl again to treat yourself to a soothing, enriching facial by whipping up your own mask recipes right from the ingredients in your kitchen cupboards, refrigerator or garden.

Kick your feet up and enjoy a relaxing, skin rejuvenating treat. What the heck, close your eyes and add two used green tea bags or slices of cucumber over those tired eyes for a totally decadent experience.

* SKINSATIONAL TIP:

On average, skin cells turn over every 30 days so treat yourself to an exfoliating facial treatment at least once a month!

~ Skin Enriching Mask ~

- 1 tablespoon honey
- 1 egg yolk
- 1/2 teaspoon olive oil
- 1 tablespoon yogurt

Whisk the honey, egg yolk and yogurt together thoroughly. Slowly drizzle in the olive oil while whisking briskly.

Apply to skin for 15 to 20 minutes. Rinse well with warm water.

~ Pawpaw Vitamin Rich Facial Mask ~

- 1/2 ripe pawpaw
- 1 packet of unflavored gelatin
- 1 egg

Mash the ripe pawpaw then mix in one packet of unflavored gelatin. Lightly beat the egg and add to the pawpaw mixture blending until smooth.

Apply for 15 to 20 minutes. Rinse well with warm water.

---

* SKINSATIONAL TIP:

Although the PawPaw is not widely known outside of its particular growing region, the properties of this fruit are considered highly effective in the treatment of acne outbreaks.

~ Chocolate Facial Mask Recipe ~

- 1/3 cup cocoa
- 1/4 cup of honey
- 2 tablespoons of heavy cream or sour cream
- 3 teaspoons of oatmeal

Combine all ingredients then mix together thoroughly.

Apply to the skin by gently massaging in a slow upwards sweeping motion so that the oatmeal will exfoliate the dead skin cell layer.

Let set for 20 minutes. Rinse well with warm water.

* * *

~ Soothing Sensations ~

- 1/4 cup plain yogurt
- 2 tablespoons fresh aloe vera gel
- 2 tablespoons rose petals
- 1 tablespoon honey

Finely chopped the rose petals then squeeze the gel from the aloe vera leaves. Combine all ingredients then mix together well.

Gently massage into skin and let set for 15 minutes. Rinse well with warm water.

* * *

~ Peaches and Cream ~

- 1 ripe peach
- 1/2 lemon
- 1/2 cup light cream
- 3 to 5 springs of fresh mint
- 1/8 cup cornmeal

Into a small sauce pan add the cornmeal. Roughly cut the peach into cubes, removing the pit. Grate the rind and squeeze the juice from the lemon. Finely chop the mint leaves. Combine all ingredients with the cream into the sauce pan.

Simmer over medium low heat, stirring occasionally until the peach is completely soft and mushy. Mash the mixture into a very smooth paste.

Cool slightly and apply the warm mask to the skin for 15 minutes. Rinse well with warm water.

* * *

~ Rejuvenating Mask ~

- 2 teaspoons plain yogurt
- 1/2 teaspoon honey
- 1/2 teaspoon fresh lemon juice
- 4 to 6 grapes

Add all ingredients to a mini food processor and pulse until thoroughly pureed.

Apply a thin, even layer to the skin. Let set for 20 to 25 minutes. Rinse well with warm water.

* * *

~ Blueberry Bliss ~

- 1/4 cup fresh blueberries
- 1 tablespoon honey

- 2 tablespoons freshly squeezed lemon juice
- 2 teaspoons cornstarch

Pulse all ingredients together in a food processor until a smooth creamy paste forms.

Apply to skin and let absorb for 20 minutes. Rinse well with warm water.

* SKINSATIONAL TIP:

Gently apply skin care treatments in an upwards sweeping motion from the bottom center of each side of your face to the top outer areas. After rinsing, gently tap the surface of the skin repeatedly to stimulate circulation.

~ *Cleopatra's Silky Secret* ~

- 1/2 cup heavy cream
- 1/2 cup rose hips
- 1/2 cup rose petals
- 1/4 cup oatmeal

Finely chop the rose hips and rose petals in a food processor. Add the cream and chopped roses to a small saucepan. Gently simmer over medium low heat for 10 minutes. Slowly stir in enough of the oatmeal to thicken into a smooth paste.

Gently massage onto skin. Leave on for up to 30 minutes. Rinse well with warm water.

* * *

~ Hydrating Facial Mask ~

- 1 egg yolk
- 1/2 avocado
- drizzle of cider vinegar

Whisk the egg yolk until light and foamy. Thoroughly mash the avocado drizzling in enough cider vinegar to form a soft, smooth paste. Whisk the avocado mixture into the egg yolk.

Apply a thin layer and let set for 15 to 20 minutes. Rinse well with warm water.

* * *

~ Skin Firming Mask ~

- 1/2 lemon
- 1 egg white
- 1/2 packet unflavored gelatin
- 1 tablespoon of cornstarch

Using a mixer, whip the egg white until stiff peaks form. Sprinkle in the cornstarch and gelatin. Continue to beat the mixture together on the lowest mixer speed until combined. Add the juice of the half of lemon and mix together well.

Apply a thin layer and let set for 20 minutes. Rinse well with warm water.

* SKINSATIONAL TIP:

Gelatin is made from collagen taken from the connective tissue of animals. Gelatin helps facial peels to set and serves to tighten the skin which encourages the reduction of pore size.

~ Anti-Aging Mask ~

- 1 egg yolk
- 2 tablespoons of milk
- 1 teaspoon of honey
- 1 tablespoon fennel
- 1 teaspoon fresh thyme

Add all ingredients to a mini food processor and pulse until thoroughly combined.

Apply a thin, even layer to the skin. Let set for 15 minutes. Rinse well with warm water.

~ Moisturizing Mask ~

- 3 tablespoons plain yogurt
- 2 tablespoons oatmeal
- 1 teaspoon natural raw sugar
- 1 tablespoon honey

Cook the oatmeal according to the directions on the package using the yogurt instead of water. Mix in the sugar and honey. Allow the mixture to cool slightly.

Apply the warm mixture for 10 to 15 minutes. Rinse well with warm water.

* * *

~ Face Firming Mask ~

- 1 tablespoon of honey
- 1 tablespoon of freshly squeezed orange juice
- 1 tablespoon of cream of tartar
- 1 egg white

In a bowl whisk the egg white until light and frothy then slowly sprinkle in the cream of tartar a little at a time while continuing to whisk briskly. Add the honey and orange juice and whisk again until all ingredients are incorporated.

Place the mixture in the microwave for 30 seconds to warm. Apply a thin layer of the warm mixture to the skin to the face and throat.

Let set for 15 minutes or until the mixture begins to dry. Rinse completely with warm water.

* * *

~ Soothing, Healing Mask ~

- 1/8 cup buttermilk
- 2 tablespoon aloe vera gel
- 2 teaspoons honey
- 1 tablespoon rosemary leaves
- 2 tablespoons tapioca

Express the aloe gel from 2 to 3 large leaves. Finely mince the rosemary leaves. Combine all ingredients and mix well. Let the mixture rest for at least 10 minutes prior to use.

Apply for 15 minutes. Rinse well with warm water.

* * *

~ Dry Skin Mask ~

- 1/4 cup dry powdered milk
- 1 egg yolk
- 1 teaspoon honey
- 1/4 cup oatmeal
- 1/8 cup mineral water
- 1/2 tablespoon green tea leaves

In a small saucepan cook the oatmeal according to package directions using mineral water and tea leaves. Cool slightly then whisk in the honey followed by the egg yolk then the powdered milk.

Apply the warm mixture for 15 minutes. Rinse well with warm water.

---

* SKINSATIONAL TIP:

The more potent beneficial properties of fruits such as the tomato and peach are found in the skin of the fruit.

~ Moisture Pack ~

- 1 tablespoon sunflower oil
- 1/4 avocado
- 2 tablespoons banana
- 2 lavender flowers

Finely chop the lavender flowers. Thoroughly mash the banana and avocado. Mix in the lavender flowers. Slowly add in the sunflower oil while continuing to mix the ingredients until a smooth paste forms.

Apply for 10 minutes. Rinse well with warm water.

~ Batter Up ~

- 1 egg white
- 2 tablespoons grapefruit juice
- 1 teaspoon licorice root
- 1 tablespoon cornstarch

Whip the egg white into stiff peaks. Finely grate the licorice root and then juice a large wedge of grapefruit. Add all the ingredients to the egg white and whip together until thoroughly combined.

Apply for 20 minutes. Rinse well with warm water.

* * *

~ Enriching Egg Mask ~

- 1 tablespoon mango
- 1/2 teaspoon olive oil
- 1 tablespoon sour cream
- 1 tablespoon soy flour
- 1 egg

Whip egg until frothy then puree the mango in a blender. Add all ingredients to the egg mixture and beat until all ingredients are combined.

Apply for 15 to 20 minutes. Rinse well with warm water.

~ Miracle Facial Whip ~

- 1/4 cup Miracle Whip
- 2 tablespoons orange juice
- 1 tablespoon honey

Whisk all ingredients together until thoroughly combined.

Gently massage into skin. Let set for 20 to 30 minutes. Rinse well with warm water.

* * *

~ Grapefruit Delight ~

- 1 egg white
- 2 tablespoons cornstarch
- 1 tablespoon cream of tartar
- 1/4 cup grapefruit juice
- 1 teaspoon coarse sea salt

Beat cornstarch, cream of tartar and salt into egg whites until glossy. Slowly add the freshly squeezed grapefruit juice.

Apply generously and let set for 15 minutes. Rinse well with warm water.

~ Chocolate Decadence ~

- 1/3 cup cocoa powder
- 1/4 cup honey
- 2 tablespoons heavy cream
- 3 teaspoons rolled oats

Mix all ingredients together thoroughly.

Gently massage into skin and let set for 20 minutes. Rinse well with lukewarm water.

* SKINSATIONAL TIP:

Using the dry brush exfoliation technique before or after a home facial helps to remove flaking and dead skin cells as well as stimulates circulation.

~ Tropical Paradise ~

- 1/2 passion fruit
- 2 tablespoons dark cocoa powder
- 1 tablespoon coconut oil
- 1 tablespoon coconut milk

Pulse all ingredients together in food processor until thick and smooth.

Apply to skin and let set for 25 minutes. Rinse well with warm water.

* * *

~ Rejuvenating Wonder ~

- 1/2 tablespoon honey
- 2 tablespoons plain yogurt
- 1 tablespoon lime juice
- 2 to 3 fresh sage leaves
- 5 plain generic brand aspirin
- 3 to 5 mashed grapes

Finely crush the aspirin tablets. Add all ingredients to a blender and puree all ingredients together thoroughly.

Apply for 15 to 20 minutes. Rinse well with warm water.

* * *

~ Moisturizing Magic ~

- 1/8 cup soy powder
- 1/2 apricot
- 2 tablespoons heavy cream
- 1 tablespoon honey
- 3 fresh mint leaves

Finely chop the mint and remove the pit from the apricot. Combine all ingredients into a food processor and pulse until well combined.

Gently massage into skin. Let set for 20 minutes. Rinse well with warm water.

* * *

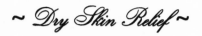

~ *Dry Skin Relief* ~

- 1/4 cup silken tofu
- 1 egg yolk
- 1 tablespoon buttermilk
- 1 tablespoon honey
- 1 lettuce leaf

Puree all ingredients together in a blender until thick and creamy.

Apply to skin and let set 20 minutes. Rinse well with warm water.

* SKINSATIONAL TIP:

Lettuce has a rich herbal lore history as a treatment for bruising and mild skin adhesions due to analgesic properties. It is also used as a natural eyewash remedy to treat eye irritations such as conjunctivitis.

~ Sinfully Soft & Simple ~

- 1 ounce dark chocolate
- 2 to 3 teaspoons buttermilk
- 2 tablespoons raw sugar

Melt the chocolate in microwave for 30 seconds. Combine well with remaining ingredients.

Gently massage into skin and let set 10 minutes. Rinse well with warm water.

* * *

~ Banana Bonanza ~

- 1/2 ripe banana
- 1 1/2 tablespoons orange juice
- 1 heaping tablespoon raw sugar
- 1 tablespoon corn syrup

Mash the banana then combine freshly squeezed orange juice, corn syrup, and sugar to form a smooth paste.

Apply to skin for 15 minutes. Rinse well with warm water.

~ The Princess and the Tea ~

- 3 to 5 green tea bags
- 1/3 cup vitamin water (found in the spring water aisle in grocery markets and variety stores)
- 1 egg white
- 1 tablespoon lemon juice
- 1 tablespoon cornstarch

Add the tea bags to boiling vitamin water and let tea bags steep until cool. Meanwhile, whisk the egg white until frothy. Add the lemon juice and cornstarch while continuing to whisk briskly. Squeeze the tea bags into the mixture then slowly mix in the cooled tea.

Apply a thin layer to skin and let set 20 minutes. Rinse with lukewarm water.

* * *

~ Tomato Twist ~

- 2 tablespoons coarse sea salt
- 2 small tomatoes
- 1 tablespoon rosemary
- 2 teaspoons extra virgin olive oil

Dice the tomatoes and finely chop the rosemary. Add all ingredients to a sauce pan and let simmer over low heat until reduced by half. Let cool slightly. Use a blender to process mixture until smooth.

Apply to skin while still warm for 15 minutes. Rinse well with warm water.

* * *

~ Strawberry Delight ~

- 3 to 5 strawberries
- 3 tablespoons dry powdered milk
- 2 tablespoons almond or walnut oil

Process all ingredients together in a mini-food processor until smooth.

Apply to skin for 15 to 20 minutes. Rinse well with warm water.

~ Facial Peels ~

Natural skincare facial peels are an excellent way to promote the rejuvenation of aging skin.

However, skin peels are typically viewed as a more aggressive strategy for treating aging skin and are usually not recommended to be used more than once a week.

Many recipes for natural skincare peels typically utilize fruit acids because of their exfoliating properties in addition to a skin tightening ingredient such as gelatin or egg whites.

Occasional facial peels are great for the skin because they loosen dead skin cells which improve the texture of the skin while restoring elasticity, reducing pore size, diminishing fine lines and wrinkles, minimizing hyperpigmentation as well as stimulating collagen production.

Natural skin care peels also help to transform tired, dull appearing skin leaving the face extremely soft, smooth, more vibrant. Peels, or nearly any other skin treatment for that matter, are the most effective when the skin is the most receptive. Apply a skin peel treatment right after a short facial steam while the skin is still warm and moist.

~ *Acne Blaster* ~

- 5 plain aspirin tablets
- 5 pot marigold (calendula) flowers
- 1 egg white

Finely grind the plain aspirin tablets, (a coffee grinder or mortar and pestle works quite well). Finely chop the marigold flowers. Beat the egg white in a mixer until thick and foamy. Add the marigold flowers and aspirin tablets and mix again until all ingredients are thoroughly combined.

Apply to skin for 15 to 20 minutes until set. Rinse well with warm water.

~ Comfy Comfrey Peel ~

- 1/2 cup comfrey leaves
- 2 tablespoons cider vinegar
- 1/4 cup parsley
- 2 tablespoons cornstarch
- 1 tablespoon cream of tartar

Pulse ingredients in food processor until well incorporated drizzling in enough of the cider vinegar to create a smooth paste.

Apply a thin layer to skin for 20 minutes. Rinse well with warm water.

* * *

~ Razzle Dazzle Raspberry ~

- 1/4 cup raspberries
- 1 tablespoon plain yogurt
- 1 packet unflavored gelatin
- 2 fresh mint leaves
- 1 ice cube

Whip all ingredients together in a blender until smooth and thick.

Apply for 15 minutes. Rinse well with warm water.

~ The Banana Peel ~

- 1/4 small banana
- 1 egg white
- 1 tablespoon cornstarch

Thoroughly mash the banana then whip the egg white with the cornstarch until stiff. Slowly add the banana and mix until completely incorporated.

Apply a thin layer to the face and let set for up to 30 minutes. Rinse completely with warm water.

* * *

~ Skin Firming Peel ~

- 1 packet unflavored gelatin
- 1 lemon
- 1 orange
- 1 stalk rhubarb

Finely grate the rind from the lemon and orange into a small saucepan. Roughly chop the rhubarb. Add the juice from both fruits and the rhubarb to the saucepan then heat mixture over very low heat until rhubarb is thoroughly cooked. Let cool slightly, add gelatin then puree mixture in a blender.

Apply warm mixture to skin for 15 minutes. Rinse well with warm water.

* SKINSATIONAL TIP:

The medicinal attributes of rhubarb date back to ancient Chinese civilizations. Rhubarb is a powerful astringent with antioxidant and cleansing properties.

~ Gentle Fruit Peel ~

- 1 cup fresh pineapple
- 1/2 cup fresh papaya
- 1 tablespoon honey
- 1 tablespoon cream of tartar

In a blender, puree the fruit together then add the honey and cream of tartar. Blend into a smooth paste.

Apply for 20 minutes. Rinse with warm water.

~ Anti-Wrinkle Peel ~

- 1/4 cucumber
- 1 egg white
- 1 teaspoon lemon juice
- 4 evening primrose blossoms
- 2 echinacea blossoms

Combine all ingredients into a food processor. Pulse until all ingredients are pureed together well.

Apply for 15 minutes. Rinse well with warm water.

* * *

~ PH Restorative Peel ~

- 1 tomato
- 1 package unflavored gelatin
- 1 tablespoon fennel
- 1 teaspoon lemongrass
- 1/2 package dry yeast

Finely grate the lemongrass then roughly chop the tomato and fennel. Combine all ingredients in a saucepan over medium low heat and simmer until the tomato is soft. Puree mixture until smooth.

Apply for 20 minutes. Rinse well with warm water.

~ Skin Revitalizing Peel ~

- 1 egg yolk
- 1 tsp honey
- 1/8 cup fresh citrus (lemon, orange or lime) juice
- 1/8 cup tapioca
- 1 packet unflavored gelatin

Whisk all ingredients until well combined.

Apply for 20 to 25 minutes. Rinse well with warm water.

* * *

~ Hydrating and Moisturizing Peel ~

- 1/4 avocado
- 1 teaspoon honey
- 1 egg white
- 4 rose hips

Mash the avocado then roughly chop the rose hips. Whip the egg white in a blender then add the remaining ingredients and mix until well combined.

Apply for 15 minutes. Rinse well with warm water.

~ Basil Balm ~

- 1/4 cup basil leaves
- 2 teaspoons baking soda
- 1 tablespoon sugar
- 1 packet plain unflavored gelatin
- 3 tablespoons wine vinegar

Roughly chop the basil leaves. Combine all ingredients in a blender and whip together until smooth.

Apply for 10 minutes. Rinse well with warm water.

* * *

~ Apple Facial Glaze ~

- 1/4 apple
- 3 tablespoons carrot
- 1/8 teaspoon nutmeg
- 2 tablespoons grapefruit juice
- 1/2 packet plain gelatin

Roughly chop the apple, grate the carrot and squeeze the juice from a large wedge of grapefruit. Place all ingredients into a small sauce pan and simmer over medium low heat until the apple begins to fall apart. Let cool slightly.

Apply warm mixture to skin for 15 minutes. Rinse well with warm water.

* SKINSATIONAL TIP:

Malic acid, a natural form of alpha hydroxyl acid, is found in apples, vinegar and cider. It is a mild exfoliant with astringent properties.

~ Sweet Potato Peel ~

- 4 dried apricots
- 1/2 sweet potato
- 2 green tea bags
- 1 cup mineral water
- 1 packet plain gelatin

Boil all ingredients except the gelatin together until soft and mushy and the liquid is reduced by half. Let cool slightly then transfer mixture to a blender, adding the gelatin. Puree until smooth and creamy.

Apply for 15 minutes. Rinse well with warm water.

~ Skin Witchery ~

- 1 tablespoon cream of tartar
- 1/8 cup witch hazel leaves and seeds
- 1/4 cup dry powdered egg whites
- 2 tablespoons pomegranate juice

Pulse the witch hazel leaves and seeds in a food processor. Add the remaining ingredients and pulse together until well mixed.

Apply for 10 minutes. Rinse well with warm water.

---

* SKINSATIONAL TIP:

Squeezing a leaf of witch hazel on an insect bite will reduce the swelling, pain and itching.

~ Pineapple Peel ~

- 1 egg white
- 1/3 cup pineapple
- 1/2 packet unflavored gelatin
- 3 tablespoons dry powdered soy protein
- 2 teaspoons sesame oil

Use a blender to whip the egg white until frothy. Add the remaining ingredients and whip again into a smooth paste.

Apply for 20 minutes. Rinse well with warm water.

~ *Heal Peel* ~

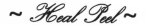

- 1 egg yolk
- 2 tablespoons aloe vera gel
- 1 lime
- 2 tablespoons cornstarch
- 1 tablespoon flax seed oil

Express the gel from 2 to 3 large aloe vera leaves. Combine all ingredients and whisk together well.

Gently massage into skin and let set for 20 minutes. Rinse well with warm water.

* * *

~ *Just Peachy Peel* ~

- 1 peach
- 1 egg white
- 3 leaves fresh mint
- 2 tablespoons baking soda
- 5 plain aspirin tablets

Crush the aspirin into a fine dust. Roughly chop the peach, removing the pit. Whip the egg white in blender until frothy then add the remaining ingredients and whip again until thoroughly pureed.

Apply for 15 minutes. Rinse well with warm water.

---

* SKINSATIONAL TIP:

Applying the juice squeezed from a new leaf of a peach tree is an effective treatment for age spots and blemishes.

~ Heavenly Power Peel ~

- 1/8 cup soy milk powder
- 2 to 3 tablespoons apricot nectar or juice
- 2 tablespoons coconut milk
- 1/8 cup dark cocoa powder

Combine all ingredients and whisk together into a smooth paste.

Gently massage into skin. Let set for 15 to 20 minutes. Rinse well with warm water.

~ Dandelion Cleansing Glaze ~

- 1/8 cup thistle tops
- 1/4 cup young dandelion leaves
- 1 grapefruit
- 2 sprigs fresh chervil
- 1 packet unflavored plain gelatin

Grate the rind from the grapefruit then squeeze the juice into a food processor. Combine all ingredients and pulse until thoroughly mixed.

Apply for 10 minutes. Rinse well with warm water.

* SKINSATIONAL TIP:

*Remove blackheads quickly and easily by mixing
equal amounts of plain gelatin with a freshly
squeezed citrus juice, dairy product or miracle whip.
Heat briefly in the microwave, apply to affected
areas and allow to dry for up to a half an hour.
Peel off then rinse well with warm water.*

~ Facial Toners ~

Using an organic skin care facial toner is an important step in any skin care regimen.

Not only is using a facial toner an excellent opportunity to introduce an anti-aging treatment into your regimen, toners also gently remove dead skin cells, excess oils, and any impurities.

Not to mention that toning gives the skin a final cleansing so it will look bright, healthy and refreshed.

Organic skin care ingredients have many rejuvenating properties that tone, firm, strengthen skin cells, hydrate, reduce pore size, repair and protect the skin.

Incorporating an anti-aging treatment as an ingredient in a natural facial toner recipe is an excellent strategy to maximize the opportunities to effectively treat aging skin and help to stimulate skin rejuvenation.

Toners help hydrate, condition and restore the skin's natural pH balance. To produce the best effects, apply facial toner to clean, warm, moist skin. Toners also help to stimulate the skin and increase the ability of moisturizers to penetrate though the layers of skin, allowing the essential properties of ingredients to absorb into the skin quickly.

Toning often leaves the skin feeling invigorated while giving the skin a healthy glow. So get out your mixing bowl and cotton balls and whisk yourself away to an organic skin care revitalizing and rejuvenating treat!

~ Flower Toning Power ~

- 1/3 cup violet blossoms
- 1/3 cup jasmine blossoms
- 1/3 cup echinecea blossoms
- 1 1/2 cup white wine vinegar

Puree all ingredients in blender. Let mixture infuse together for several hours. Strain into container.

Use to tone daily.

* SKINSATIONAL TIP:

The sun is one of the biggest culprits in drying out the skin, causing skin damage, and accelerating the aging process.

~ Got Milk? Cleansing Milk Toner ~

- 1/2 cup milk
- 5 nettle leaves
- 5 pansy blossoms
- 5 peppermint leaves

Roughly chop the nettle leaves, peppermint and pansy blossoms. Combine all ingredients in a small bottle and let infuse overnight.

Lightly saturate a cotton ball or cosmetic pad to cleanse and tone the skin daily. Store in the refrigerator for up to one week.

* * *

~ Mix and Match Fruit Acid Toners ~

- Juice one or several citrus fruits: lemon, lime, orange and/or grapefruit
- Select one or several herbs to infuse the fruit acid: rosemary, sage, thyme, mint, or marjoram and/or
- Select one or several medicinal flowers: witch hazel seeds, elder, yarrow, chamomile, comfrey, rose blossoms and/or rose hips

Combine all your selected ingredients into a sterile squeeze bottle and let set for several hours to allow the ingredients to marinate.

As an alternative, simply squeeze the juice from any of the fruits listed, saturate a cotton ball and swab the surface of the skin. It's simple, quick, easy and effective with no mixing involved!

This is a great recipe to use your creativity!

Mix and match the variety of herbs and ingredients to infuse the citrus juice. The fruit acid toners can be refrigerated and used for up to one week.

* SKINSATIONAL TIP:

The antioxidant mechanisms in vitamins such as A, C, and E as well as the retinoid derivatives of vitamin A help to reduce skin damage caused by free radicals.

~ *Restoration* ~

- 1 cup soy milk
- 1 1/2 tablespoons baking soda
- 2 tablespoons almonds
- 1/2 small beet
- 1 small potato

Grind the almonds into a fine powder in a coffee grinder. Finely grate the potato and beet, skin and all. Combine all ingredients into a small saucepan and simmer over medium low heat for 20 minutes. Let cool completely.

Press mixture through a sieve, straining into bottle and store in the refrigerator.

Use to tone skin daily.

* * *

~ *Peppermint Potion* ~

- 1/2 cup soy milk
- 1/2 cup nasturtium flowers
- 1/8 cup fresh peppermint leaves

Blend all ingredients together well in a food processor. Let mixture infuse for several hours then strain into a clean, sterile container.

Use to tone skin daily.

* * *

~ *Papaya Toning Perfection* ~

- 1 papaya
- 1/2 cup red wine vinegar
- 1 teaspoon sea salt

Roughly chop the papaya then place all ingredients into a small saucepan and simmer together over low heat for 30 to 45 minutes stirring occasionally. Set mixture aside to cool completely.

Strain liquid into small bottle. Use daily to tone and condition the skin.

* SKINSATIONAL TIP:

Enzymes found in many fruits and plants such as pumpkin, pineapple and papaya are excellent natural exfoliants that work to effectively dissolve dead skin cells.

~ Toning Transformations ~

- 1/2 cup elder buds; flowers and/or berries
- 2 lemons
- 2 teaspoons raw sugar

Roughly chop the elder berries and /or flowers. Grate the rind from both the lemons then juice lemons. Combine all ingredients into clean, sterile jar. Shake well and let ingredients infuse for several hours. Strain prior to use.

Use mixture to tone skin daily.

~ *Rapid Recovery* ~

- gel from 3 large aloe leaves
- 3 sprigs rosemary
- 2 sage leaves
- 1/8 cup light cream

Express the gel from the aloe leaves. Finely mince the rosemary and sage leaves. Whisk all ingredients together well and refrigerate overnight. Strain into small container.

Use to gently tone skin daily.

* * *

~ *Tea Thyme Toner* ~

- 5 sprigs thyme
- 1 sprig sage
- 2 chamomile tea bags
- 2 green tea bags
- 2 cups mineral water

Brew all ingredients together in a small saucepan on medium heat for 10 minutes. Let cool completely. Squeeze the liquid from the tea bags back into the saucepan. Strain into small bottle.

Use toner once daily.

~ *Mimosa Magic* ~

- 1/8 cup champagne vinegar
- 1 orange

Grate the rind from the orange then squeeze the juice into a small container. Add the vinegar and shake well. Let the ingredients infuse for several hours prior to use.

Saturate cotton ball to tone skin daily.

> ## * SKINSATIONAL TIP:
>
> *The tartaric and citric acid properties of natural apple cider, fermented fruit, coconut and rice vinegars have a wide range of rejuvenating attributes.*

~ *Rosemary Astringent* ~

- 5 plain generic aspirin
- 4 sprigs rosemary leaves
- 1/8 cup witch hazel seeds
- 1/4 cup cider vinegar

Finely crush the aspirin tablets then add them to a food processor with the remaining ingredients. Pulse together until thoroughly mixed. Strain into bottle.

Use to tone acne prone skin daily.

* * *

~ The Dynamic Duo ~

- 1 cup coconut cream
- 1 cup lavender flowers

Puree ingredients in blender. Let mixture infuse for several hours before straining into small container.

Use to tone dry, sensitive skin daily.

* * *

~ Pumpkin Spice ~

- 1 1/2 cups vitamin water
- 1/2 cup pumpkin
- 1/4 teaspoon nutmeg
- 1/8 cup fresh cranberries

Peel, then finely dice the pumpkin. Add all ingredients in small saucepan and simmer together over medium low heat until the pumpkin and cranberries are mushy.

Mash together then press through sieve straining mixture into a container.

Use as daily toning treatment.

~ Tomato Skin Tonic ~

- 1/4 cup cider vinegar
- 1 tomato
- 1 tablespoon epsom salts

Roughly chop the tomato then add all ingredients into a blender. Puree until smooth. Strain into container.

Use to tone skin daily.

* * *

~ Carrot Conditioning Toner ~

- 2 carrots
- 3 tablespoons ginger root
- 1 tablespoon marjoram
- 1 1/4 cups almond milk

Finely dice the carrots and add to a small saucepan. Simmer ingredients together over medium heat until carrots are thoroughly cooked. Press mixture through a sieve, straining into a container. Store in the refrigerator for up to one week.

Use as daily toning treatment.

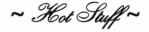
~ Hot Stuff ~

- 1/2 cup mineral water
- 2 tablespoons apricot tea leaves
- 2 tablespoons black tea leaves
- 1 lime
- 5 cranberries

Grate the rind from the lime then squeeze the juice from the lime into a small saucepan. Simmer all ingredients over medium low heat for 20 to 25 minutes.

Cool completely then press mixture through a sieve, straining into microwave safe container.

Briefly heat the toner in the microwave prior to using each morning.

---

* SKINSATIONAL TIP:

The herb rosemary has a long history in herbal lore as a natural astringent with antibacterial properties. It also stimulates circulation as well as treats a variety of skin conditions including acne and restoring elasticity to the skin.

~ Facial Steams ~

Facial steaming is a great strategy to incorporate into any skin care routine and should be considered a fundamental for addressing aging skin concerns.

Facial steaming using just a few natural ingredients just once a week is a quick and easy way to help the skin in a variety of ways including:

- *Open up and unclog pores to facilitate deep cleansing*
- *Stimulate the skin's natural process of detoxification*
- *Improve circulation and relax facial muscles*
- *Provide moisture to deeply hydrate the skin*

The process can be as simple as adding a few herbs to a bowl of steaming hot water, positioning your face over the bowl, and arranging a towel over your head so the steam doesn't escape for five to ten minutes. Home spa facial steamers are also a nice option.

Most home spa facial saunas or steamers have a temperature adjustment, a water tank that will accommodate the ingredients of any steaming recipe, and a comfortable shield that directs the steam allowing a place to rest your face during the steaming process.

Quickly cleanse the skin prior to steaming and follow with a gentle scrub to exfoliate any remaining dead skin cells and debris as well as to ensure that the pores are thoroughly cleansed. Adding a facial mask or facial peel to the weekly steaming routine will provide further nourishment and enhance the health of the skin.

* SKINSATIONAL TIP:

During the winter using a humidifier in your home as well as in your office will help keep your skin hydrated by keeping moisture in the air.

~ *Steaming Herbal Healer* ~

- 3 cups mineral water
- 1 tablespoon each of fresh fennel, oregano, thyme, rosemary, mint and sage

Finely chop all the herbs and add all ingredients to a large microwave safe container. Microwave on high until the mixture reaches a boil.

Let cool slightly prior to using as a steaming facial.

~ Citrus Blast ~

- 4 cups vitamin water
- 2 tablespoons apricot tea leaves
- 1 lime
- 1 passion fruit
- 1 grapefruit

Roughly dice the lime, passion fruit and grapefruit. Combine all ingredients into a large sauce pan. Bring to a boil for several minutes.

Turn off heat and allow to cool slightly before using as a facial steam.

* * *

~ Steamy Rose Water ~

- 1 1/2 cups soy milk
- 1/2 cup rose hips
- 1/4 cup almonds

Roughly chop the rose hips and almonds. Combine all ingredients into a large saucepan. Bring to boil for several minutes.

Turn off heat and allow to cool slightly before using as a facial steam.

* SKINSATIONAL TIP:

Rose hips are rich in vitamin C, vitamin E, B-complex vitamins, bioflavonoid, manganese and pectin.

~ Coconut Facial Brew ~

- 1 cup fresh coconut milk
- 1 tablespoon ginger root
- 1/4 cup blackberries

Roughly chop the blackberries. Finely grate the ginger root then combine all ingredients in a small saucepan and simmer slowly over medium low heat for 15 minutes.

Remove from heat and let cool slightly prior to steaming.

* * *

~ Dream Steam ~

- 3 green tea bags
- 5 sprigs fresh spearmint

- small bunch of lemongrass
- 1 teaspoon sesame oil
- 1 quart water

Microwave all ingredients together until just boiling in a small microwave safe bowl.

Let cool slightly before facial steaming.

* * *

~ Hot Lavender Mist ~

- 1 sprig rosemary
- 1/3 cup lavender flowers
- 2 cups mineral water
- 2 teaspoons mineral oil

Finely chop the rosemary and lavender. Combine all ingredients in small saucepan set over medium high heat until the mixture just begins to boil.

Remove from heat and let cool slightly prior to steaming.

* * *

~ Some Like It Hot ~

- 2 cups milk
- 2 carrots
- 1/8 cup fennel
- 1 tablespoon sage

- 1 tablespoon parsley
- 2 tablespoons honey

Roughly chop the carrots, fennel and herbs. Combine all ingredients into a small saucepan. Bring to boil for several minutes.

Remove from heat and let cool slightly prior to steaming.

* SKINSATIONAL TIP:

Since the skin is the first place that is apt to exhibit symptoms of stress and anxiety be sure to create a positive outlet for those highly stressful days. A balanced diet, exercise and plenty of rest are the foundation to build upon when identifying a productive release for anxiety and stress.

~ *Facial Mists* ~

Facial Mists re-hydrate the skin on hot summer days as well as on those cold, dry, windy winter days. One of the chronic conditions of aging skin is the rapid depletion of moisture. As a result, proper hydration is an essential cornerstone in any anti-aging skin care routine for maintaining skin health.

Spritzing the skin with a natural fortified mist of nutrients helps to rebalance moisture levels, provide the skin with additional antioxidants, and essential nourishment. These facial rejuvenation natural recipes are formulated with ingredients that stimulate cell repair, renewal and help protect the skin from free radical damage.

Keep a small misting bottle of your favorite skin spritz recipe in your car, at your office, in your beach bag and in your purse for a quick light and refreshing "pick-me-up" for tired, dull looking skin throughout the day!

* SKINSATIONAL TIP:

Keep your skin hydrated inside and out by drinking at least 6 to 8 glasses of water a day. The more moisture your body loses, the more you need to drink in order to replenish the water content in your body.

~ Basic Rose Water Misting Spray ~

- 1 cup rose flowers
- 1 cup rose hips
- 2 cups mineral water

Finely chop rose petals and rose hips in a food processor. Combine all ingredients in a small saucepan and simmer over low medium heat for 30 minutes.

Let cool completely. Press mixture through sieve while straining into a small misting spray bottle.

Use to mist face throughout the day.

---

* SKINSATIONAL TIP:

Rose hips and rose petals are a versatile skin rejuvenation ingredient and are very effective in treating a variety of aging skin conditions. Soak cotton balls in the rose misting solution and pop in the freezer to reduce under eye puffiness.

~ Mint Mist ~

- 1 tablespoon barley

- 1/4 cup fresh mint
- 2 cups vitamin water
- I/2 teaspoon honey

Combine all ingredients into a blender and mix thoroughly. Strain mixture into a small misting bottle.

Use to liberally to mist skin throughout the day.

* * *

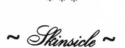

~ *Skinsicle* ~

- 3 to 4 chamomile tea bags
- 2 cups water
- 1 teaspoon mineral oil
- 1 tablespoon ginger root
- 1/4 cup jasmine flower blossoms

Grate the ginger root then finely chop the jasmine blossoms into a small saucepan. Add the remaining ingredients and bring mixture to a simmer for 15 to 20 minutes.

Let cool completely before squeezing out the tea bags back into the pot. Strain mixture into a small misting bottle. Place in the freezer for up to one hour.

Use to mist face frequently throughout the day.

~ *Moisturizing Mist* ~

- 2 cups vitamin water
- 1/4 cup soy milk powder
- 2 tablespoons rosemary
- 1/3 cup rose hips

Pulse dry ingredients in food processor until finely chopped. Combine all ingredients into a small saucepan over medium low heat and simmer together for 20 minutes.

Let mixture cool before straining into mist bottle.

Use to mist face several times a day.

* * *

~ *Lavender Spritz* ~

- 1/4 cup lavender blossoms
- 1 tablespoon coconut oil
- 1/8 cup green tea leaves
- 2 cups mineral water
- 2 sprigs fresh spearmint

Finely chop the lavender blossoms and spearmint. Add all ingredients to a small saucepan and simmer over medium low heat for up to 30 minutes.

Let cool completely before pressing ingredients through a sieve to strain mixture into a small misting bottle. Place into the freezer for up to one hour.

Use to mist face frequently throughout the day.

* * *

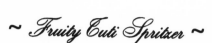

~ *Fruity Tuti Spritzer* ~

- 1 orange
- 1 apple
- 1 lime
- 2 cups vitamin water

Grate the rind from the orange and lime then squeeze the juice from both fruits into a small saucepan. Roughly chop the apple along with what remains of the orange and lime. Add all ingredients to the saucepan and simmer over medium low until the apple becomes soft.

Let cool completely before pressing mixture through a sieve to strain into a small misting bottle.

Use to mist face several times throughout the day.

* * *

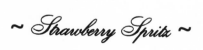

~ *Strawberry Spritz* ~

- 1 grapefruit
- 1 lime

- 1/2 cup strawberries
- 1 1/2 cups skim milk

Roughly chop the grapefruit, lime and strawberries then add all ingredients to a small saucepan. Simmer ingredients together over medium low heat for 20 to 30 minutes.

Let cool completely before pressing mixture through a sieve to strain into a small misting bottle.

Use to mist face several times throughout the day.

* * *

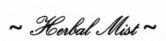
~ Herbal Mist ~

- 1 1/2 cups coconut milk
- 1 tablespoon each sage, thyme, marjoram
- 4 black tea bags
- 1 tablespoon ginger root

Grate the ginger root into a small saucepan. Combine all remaining ingredients and let simmer over medium low heat for 20 minutes.

Let cool completely. Squeeze tea bags back into the mixture before pressing through a sieve to strain into a small misting bottle.

Use to mist face several times throughout the day.

~ Facial Cleansers ~

Facial Cleansers are a critical element in any natural skin care routine in order to keep your skin healthy. Finding the right one for your skin type is not only the first but the most important step in your skin care regimen.

By now it isn't a surprise to learn that soaps, especially those with detergents or chemicals, are very harsh and will only dry out the skin. Soaps tend to strip the natural oils from the skin and can destroy the barriers that serve to protect the skin from daily exposure to the elements. A face wash that is homemade is a much gentler and affordable option.

Not only does washing your face remove dead skin cells, oil build up, dissolve impurities and the small particles of dirt that collect on the surface of the skin but cleansing the skin also improves circulation, protects against break-outs and stimulates skin cell renewal.

Of course, we all know that younger skin generates cell renewal much faster than older skin which makes carefully caring for aging skin all that more important.

Who knew you could accomplish so much by simply washing your face?

Selecting an appropriate facial cleanser for your skin type is essential. Although for any skin type, the gentler the face wash the better. For example, if your skin tends to be dry, make a natural facial cleanser rich in emollients.

* SKINSATIONAL TIP:

Natural skin care cleanser recipes do not typically include a foaming agent. Simply add a small amount of a rich emollient based face wash such as Aveeno soy based cleanser or a Burt Bee's natural facial cleanser to create a foaming action.

Oily skin types will want to lean towards a facial cleanser that has an acid base such as a citrus ingredient while sensitive skin types will benefit from the healing properties provided by aloe vera and green tea.

Making your own natural facial cleansers ensures that the daily build–up of debris is gently washed away without stripping away the skin's essential natural attributes. To maximize the benefits of using a natural facial cleanser, apply your homemade recipe to warm moist skin.

Use an upwards circular motion to gently massage the skin with the cleanser, then rinse well. This face wash strategy will ensure a deep cleansing of clogging debris from the pores which will leave the skin ultra clean, soft and supple.

Gently pat away the excess moisture, *never wipe*, because over time this can stretch the tissue which inevitably lead to sagging skin and those dreaded wrinkles.

Ready to get mixing?

~ Very Violet Wash ~

- 1/8 cup violet blossoms
- 2 tablespoons almonds
- 1/4 cup condensed milk

Whip all ingredients together in a blender until creamy.

Gently massage into skin. Rinse well with warm water.

---

* SKINSATIONAL TIP:

Make your own cleansing cloths by soaking large cosmetic pads in the cleanser solution, squeeze out all excess liquid and allow to dry on an absorbent paper towel. Store the cleansing pads in the refrigerator for up to 5 days.

~ Fruit Cleansing Whip ~

- 1/4 cup fresh papaya
- 1/4 cup fresh mango
- 1 tablespoon fresh thyme
- 1 egg white

Roughly chop the papaya and mango. Remove the thyme leaves from the stem. Combine all ingredients into blender and whip ingredients together until frothy.

Massage into skin to gently cleanse. Rinse well with warm water.

* * *

~ *Peachy Clean Facial* ~

- 2 ripe peaches
- 1 lemon
- 1/8 cup fresh mint
- 1 tablespoon rosemary
- 1/2 cup almond milk

Roughly chop the mint, rosemary, lemon and peaches; removing the pits from the peaches. Combine all ingredients in a small saucepan. Simmer over medium low heat until the mixture is completely soft and mushy. Mash into a very smooth, thin paste.

Cool until just barely warm. Apply liberally to cleanse skin. Rinse completely with warm water.

* * *

~ *Minty Fresh Face Wash* ~

- 1/4 cup fresh mint leaves
- 1 tablespoon kosher or sea salt
- 1/8 cup soy milk

Mix all ingredients thoroughly in a blender.

Apply to facial skin in a circular motion. Rinse well with warm water.

* * *

~ Dry Skin Cleanser ~

- 1/4 cucumber
- 1/4 cup plain yogurt
- 2 to 3 tablespoons oatmeal
- 1 teaspoon mineral oil

Peel and roughly chop the cucumber. Cook the oatmeal until done using the yogurt as the liquid. Add the remaining ingredients and simmer over medium low for 10 minutes. Puree the mixture in a blender until smooth.

Apply to facial skin in a circular motion. Rinse well with warm water.

* * *

~ Generic Cleanser ~

(All Skin Types)

- 1/8 cup almonds
- 2 tablespoons milk or light cream
- 2 teaspoon lemon juice
- 1 teaspoon lemon rind

Finely grind the almonds in a coffee grinder. Grate the rind from the lemon then squeeze the juice into a small mixing bowl. Combine all ingredients thoroughly.

Apply to facial skin in a circular motion. Rinse well with warm water.

* * *

~ *Rejuvenating Cleanser* ~

- 2 chamomile tea bags
- 1/3 cup coconut milk
- 2 tablespoons cornmeal
- 1 tablespoon plain yogurt

Combine all ingredients in a small sauce pan and simmer over medium low heat for 15 to 20 minutes. Let cool slightly. Squeeze the liquid from the tea bags into the mixture.

Apply warm cleanser to facial skin in a circular motion. Rinse well with warm water.

* * *

~ *Moisturizing Honey Wash* ~

- 1 tablespoon bran powder
- 2 tablespoons honey
- 1 teaspoon cream
- 1/8 cup rose petals

Finely dice the rose petals and place all ingredients in a microwave safe container. Heat the mixture in the microwave until they are just barely simmering. Stir ingredients until well blended.

Apply warm face wash to facial skin in a circular motion. Rinse well with warm water.

* * *

~ *Stimulating Citrus Cleanser* ~

- 1/2 grapefruit
- 1/2 passion fruit
- 2 teaspoons of lime rind
- 2 teaspoons cream of tartar
- 5 plain aspirin

Grate the rind from both the grapefruit and the lime then squeeze the juice from the grapefruit into a food processor. Roughly chop the passion fruit and crush the aspirin tablets. Combine all ingredients in the food processor and blend until smooth.

Apply to facial skin in a circular motion. Rinse well with warm water.

~ Revitalizing Cleanser ~

(All Skin Types)

- 1/8 cup apple
- 2 tablespoons plain yogurt
- 1 teaspoon olive oil
- 2 teaspoons orange juice

Roughly chop the apple and freshly squeeze the orange juice.
Combine ingredients in food processor until very smooth.

Apply to facial skin in a circular motion. Rinse well with warm water.

* * *

~ Moisturizing Cleanser ~

- 1 tablespoons castor oil
- 2 teaspoons cornmeal

- 4 grapes
- 2 teaspoons powdered milk

Combine all ingredients in a food processor and pulse until pureed.

Apply to facial skin in a circular motion. Rinse well with warm water.

***** SKINSATIONAL TIP:**

Lactic acid, a natural form of alpha hydroxyl acid, is a gentle exfoliant suitable for sensitive skin types found in milk products, powdered milk, sour cream, blackberries and tomatoes.

~ Heal and Protect Cleanser ~

- 1 large aloe vera leaf
- 1 slice of papaya
- 4 echinacea blossoms
- 2 evening primrose blossoms
- 1 tablespoon honey
- 1 teaspoon plain yogurt

Express the gel from the aloe vera leaf. Combine all ingredients in a food processor and mix well.

Apply to facial skin in a circular motion. Rinse well with warm water.

* * *

~ *Cucumber Cleanser* ~

- 1/4 cucumber
- 1 teaspoon peppermint
- 2 tablespoons plain yogurt
- 2 tablespoons soy powder

Peel and seed the cucumber. Add the roughly chopped cucumber with the remaining ingredients into a food processor. Pulse mixture until smooth.

Gently massage into skin. Rinse well with warm water.

* * *

~ *Kiwi Quick & Clean* ~

- 1/2 kiwi
- 2 tablespoons raw sugar
- 2 tablespoons orange juice

Peel the kiwi and in a small mixing bowl mash in into a paste. Stir in the sugar and freshly squeezed orange juice. Mix together well.

Gently massage into skin. Rinse well with warm water.

~ Cleansing Soy Cream ~

- 1/8 cup soy flour
- 2 tablespoons rolled oats
- 1 tablespoon rosemary
- 1/4 soy milk

Remove the rosemary leaves from the stem and add to a blender. Combine remaining ingredients and whip into a smooth paste.

Gently massage into skin. Rinse well with warm water.

* * *

~ Acne Correcting Wash ~

- 1/8 cup wheat germ
- 2 tablespoons baking soda
- 1 tablespoon rosemary
- 6 plain aspirin
- 1/8 cup grapefruit juice

Finely chop the fresh rosemary leaves. Grind the aspirin tablets into a powder. Combine all ingredients and mix together well.

Gently massage into skin. Rinse well with warm water.

~ *Lush Lavender Wash* ~

- 1/8 cup lavender blossoms
- 2 tablespoons almonds
- 1/8 cup condensed milk
- 1 tablespoon flax seed oil

Combine all ingredients in a food processor and pulse until smooth.

Gently massage into skin. Rinse well with warm water.

* * *

~ *Soothing Skin Cleanser* ~

- 3 tablespoons fresh aloe gel
- 5 fushia blossoms
- 2 tablespoons buttermilk
- 2 teaspoons baking soda

Express the gel from 2 to 3 large aloe vera leaves. Finely chop the fushia blossoms. Mix all ingredients together into a smooth paste.

Gently massage into skin. Rinse well with warm water.

~ *Moisturizers* ~

Moisturizing treatments made with homemade skin care recipes are a wonderfully effective way to rejuvenate aging skin.

To "moisturize" by definition literally means to add moisture. The simplest form of moisture is of course, water.

Skin that is kept well moisturized has a healthy glow while remaining soft and supple. Hydrated skin slows the signs of aging; much more so than skin that is not well cared for.

Maintaining hydrated; well moisturized skin goes a long way in preventing the skin from drying and chapping which, believe it or not, slows the aging process. The most obvious strategy in maintaining well hydrated skin starts from the inside out.

Drinking a sufficient amount of water throughout the day helps the skin preserve a necessary moisture balance. Keeping yourself well hydrated ensures nice plump skin cells which protect the skin against excessive moisture loss which, in turn, gives skin cells the best defense against drying out.

Just think of it this way; a grape is smooth and plump with nice, taut skin when it is at its peak but if it is deprived of moisture it will dry out and shrivel up into an extremely wrinkled and dried out husk. The same principle applies to your skin!

Aren't you more motivated now to begin taking better care of your skin?

Younger skin is much more resilient and typically needs less aid in retaining moisture and nourishment than older skin. Although, all skin types benefit from moisturizing in order to seal in moisture as well as to condition the skin. Aging skin especially reaps the rewards from the additional nourishment that rejuvenating homemade skin care treatments can provide.

Natural moisturizing treatments, especially for aging skin, commonly include natural oils, honey or aloe vera. Many homemade skin care recipes add the juice from a citrus fruit which offers additional conditioning via the antioxidant properties and a host of other rejuvenation attributes as well as aids in preventing outbreaks of blemishes.

As with any homemade skin care treatments, moisturizers are the most effective when applied to warm, damp skin. To maximize the absorption of the moisturizer, stimulate the skin cells by lightly tap the skin's surface after applying in an upwards, sweeping circular motion.

* SKINSATIONAL TIP:

Maintaining well hydrated skin and diminishing dryness helps the skin's overall ability to heal and protect itself.

Many of the more effective homemade skin care treatments for moisturizing the skin are very straightforward and quite simple. In fact many of the natural oils, which are emollients that can easily penetrate through the skin layers, are not only among the most popular natural skin care moisturizers but the most effective as well.

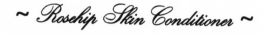

~ Rosehip Skin Conditioner ~

- 1/2 cup rosehips
- 1 lime
- 1 orange
- 2 tablespoons coconut oil

Finely chop the rosehips and place in a small sauce pan over medium low heat. Squeeze the juice from both the lime and orange over the rosehips, roughly chopping adding the remaining fruit- (skin and all) to the pan.

Simmer gently until the rosehips soften and the liquid has been reduced by half. Remove from the heat and let mixture cool slightly.

Remove lime and orange rinds before transferring mixture into a blender. Add the coconut oil. Blend until smooth adding additional freshly squeezed citrus juice if necessary.

~ Sweet Dreams Night Cream ~

- 1/2 cup almond oil
- 1 teaspoon ginger root
- 1 tablespoon sage
- 1/8 cup rose petals

Finely chop the sage and rose petals then grate the ginger root. Combine all ingredients together in a small saucepan and simmer over low heat for 20 minutes.

Let mixture steep until cool then strain into container prior to moisturizing.

* * *

~ Go Nuts! ~

Nut Oil and Natural Oil Moisturizing Options
(Especially recommended for anti-aging skin care regimens)

- Almond Oil
- Olive Oil
- Sesame Oil
- Castor Oil
- Grape Seed Oil
- Evening Primrose Oil
- Palm Oil
- Flax Seed Oil
- Peanut Oil
- Sunflower Oil
- Macadamia Oil
- Coconut Oil
- Wheat Germ Oil
- Corn Oil
- Aloe Vera Oil
- Jojoba Oil
- Avocado Oil
- Mineral Oil
- Safflower Oil
- Walnut Oil

Each oil listed is comprised of different natural properties which contribute to not only moisturizing the skin but in treating a range of aging skin issues.

Simply pick your favorite and use a small amount to gently massage into the skin in an upwards circular motion twice a day.

> ## * SKINSATIONAL TIP:
>
> *Applying skin care treatments to warm, moist skin helps the skin to thoroughly absorb all the nutrients in the treatment.*

~ Shea Facial Butter ~

- 1/8 cup shea butter
- 1 teaspoon cornstarch
- 1/8 cup rose hips
- 1/2 teaspoon safflower oil

Grind the rose hips into a fine dust. Combine all ingredients together in a mini food processor and puree until smooth. Let ingredients infuse together for several hours or overnight.

Strain into clean container prior to moisturizing. (Heat the mixture briefly in the microwave if the consistency is too thick to strain after refrigeration).

~ Velvet Aloe Vera Moisturizer ~

- 1 tablespoon flax seed oil
- 2 large aloe vera leaves

Express the aloe gel from the aloe leaves and mix together thoroughly with the flax seed oil.

Apply a light layer to the skin daily. Keep unused portion in refrigerator for up to three days.

* * *

~ Cool as a Cucumber Cream ~

- 1/8 cup walnut oil
- 1 cucumber
- 2 tablespoons fresh sage
- 2 tablespoons fresh fennel

Peel and seed the cucumber. Roughly chop the cucumber and herbs prior to combining all ingredients into a food processor. Pulse until all ingredients are mixed together well.

Let mixture infuse together for several hours or overnight.

Press through sieve into a clean container prior to moisturizing.

~ *Potpourri Lotion* ~

- 1/8 cup lavender blossoms
- 1/8 cup rose petals
- 1/8 cup nasturtium blossoms
- 1/8 cup fushia blossoms
- 1/8 cup pansy petals
- 1 cup sunflower oil

Add all flower blossoms to a food processor and pulse until finely chopped. Slowly drizzle in the sunflower oil and process until well combined. Set mixture aside for several hours or overnight in order to infuse.

Strain into clean container prior to moisturizing.

* * *

~ *Apple Berry Face Butter* ~

- 1/4 cup cranberries
- 1/2 apple
- 1/2 cup shea butter
- 1 tablespoon soy flour

Combine all ingredients together in a small saucepan over medium low heat. Gently simmer together for 25 to 30 minutes.

Use sieve to press the liquid from the mixture while straining into a container.

Use to moisturize daily.

* SKINSATIONAL TIP:

Shea butter is extracted from the shea tree which is found primarily on the African continent. It is not only a natural emollient with extensive healing properties but also provides natural UV protection from the sun.

~ Cocoa Butter Face Cream ~

- 1/4 cup cocoa butter
- 1/8 cup viola pansies
- 1 tablespoon sage
- 1 tablespoon fennel

Melt cocoa butter over very low heat. Meanwhile use a coffee grinder to finely mince the pansies and herbs prior to adding them to the cocoa butter.

Cool mixture completely prior to moisturizing. Store unused portion in the refrigerator for several days.

~ Firming Facial Fondue ~

- 1/2 cup sunflower oil
- 1/8 cup echinacea blossoms
- 1/8 cup calendula marigold petals
- 1 tablespoon licorice root

Finely chop the flower blossoms and licorice root. Combine all ingredients together in a small saucepan. Simmer over medium low heat for 20 minutes.

Let steep until cool then strain into container prior to moisturizing.

* * *

~ Skinsations ~

- 1/8 cup mineral oil
- 1 tablespoon parsley
- 1 tablespoon thyme
- 1 tablespoon lemon balm

Finely chop the herbs and combine all ingredients together in container.

Shake vigorously then let herbs infuse in the oil for several hours or overnight. Strain into a clean container prior to moisturizing.

~ Facial Wraps ~

Facial wraps are a luxurious way to indulge yourself in a wonderfully relaxing facial treatment. There are a variety of wrap mediums that range from a simple cotton cloth to more exotic options such as different kelp and seaweeds.

Facial or body wraps are utilized to help detoxify and rid the skin of impurities. The infused wrap material facilitates the skin's ability to absorb the nutrients imparted by the natural ingredients used in the recipe. Facial wraps not only stimulate circulation but also cleanse and help the skin to fortify its natural ability to heal, protect and encourage the renewal process.

The basic techniques of applying a facial wrap are very straight-forward. It is helpful to begin with wrap pieces that you have tailored and shaped to easily fit your specific facial features prior to adding the skin care mixture.

Either saturating the wrap medium with the skin care recipe solution or smoothing a thin layer of the mixture to the side of the wrap that is applied to the facial skin is all that is necessary prior to leaning back and enjoying this decadently wonderful experience.

~ Sugar Cane Exfoliating Wrap ~

- 1/4 cup sugar cane
- 2 limes
- cheesecloth

Finely grate the sugar cane and the rind from the limes. Add the freshly squeezed juice from the limes.

Soak small strips of cheesecloth in the mixture. Wring out excess liquid and position the cheesecloth strips on the cheeks, chin, nose and forehead for 15 to 20 minutes. Rinse well with warm water.

~ It's a Wrap! ~

- 1/4 cup grapes
- 1/2 orange
- 2 tablespoons honey
- 3 to 4 chamomile tea bags
- 1 cup mineral water

Puree grapes and roughly chop the orange in a food processor. Add all ingredients to a small saucepan and simmer over medium low heat for 30 minutes.

Cool slightly prior to saturating a facecloth in the mixture. Wring out excess liquid and place cloth over face for 15 minutes. Rinse well with warm water.

* * *

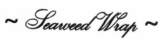

~ Seaweed Wrap ~

- nori seaweed
- 2 teaspoons each sage, fennel, marjoram
- 4 tablespoons fresh aloe gel
- 1 1/4 cups boiling water

Express the gel from 2 large aloe leaves and add half of the aloe gel to a saucepan, reserving the other half. Roughly chop the herbs and combine the aloe, herbs and water in the saucepan. Boil vigorously for several minutes.

Soak seaweed leaves in the boiling herbal water until soft and pliable. Cool slightly. Using the remaining aloe gel, apply a thin layer of the gel to one side of the nori seaweed.

Position the warm seaweed with the aloe gel side on the surface of the skin for up to 20 minutes. Rinse well with warm water.

* * *

~ Chocolate Cheese Cloth Wrap ~

- 1/4 cup dark chocolate
- 2 tablespoons fresh peppermint
- 2 to 3 tablespoons coconut milk
- Several small strips of cheesecloth

Melt chocolate slowly over very low heat. Meanwhile, finely mince the mint leaves. Stir in remaining ingredients and mix until thoroughly combined. Cool slightly.

Spread a thin layer of the warm chocolate facial mixture on small cheesecloth strips cut to fit the contours of the face.

Position the cloth strips on facial skin for 15 minutes. Rinse well with warm water.

~ Under Eye Treatments ~

Have you ever wondered why many people start to lose their vision as they age? It might just be a natural defense mechanism against creating despair as you look at yourself in the mirror and see the fine lines crinkling up around your eyes, the under eye bags that seem to get more distinctive each day or those deepening dark circles that are reminiscent of a raccoon.

There are a variety of reasons for puffy, dark under eye bags. The major reasons include fluid retention, inadequate sleep, allergies, sun damage and, of course, heredity. The puffiness is a result of the under eye area becoming a collection spot for fluids that haven't yet been absorbed into the body.

. . . .

* SKINSATIONAL TIP:

Sleeping with an extra pillow to elevate your head as high as possible while you sleep will help prevent fluids from collecting under the eye and will also help to reduce overall facial puffiness.

. . . .

Dark under eye circles are a result of tiny little capillaries and blood vessels showing through the extraordinary thin and delicate skin under the eyes. Blood deposits turn deep purple and you end up looking like you just went twelve hard rounds in a boxing ring. A poor diet, weight loss, smoking, medications that dilate blood vessels, and of course, age are all factors that contribute to those dreaded dark circles that bestow an old, tired and haggard appearance.

Specifically treating the eye area with natural ingredients will soften the fine lines, reduce swollen under eye bags and diminish dark under eye circles.

As a quick fix to reduce under eye puffiness wrap an ice cube in a soft cloth and apply to the under eye area for five minutes to reduce the swelling. Adding a very cold natural skin care treatment will also provide essential nutrients to the skin which help to heal and protect the area as well.

You should see an immediate improvement in the amount of swelling. Repeat as necessary for a few days and ~ *voila* ~ your under eye puffiness will literally vanish.

* SKINSATIONAL TIP:

Gently tapping the surface of the skin around the under eye area will help to stimulate the fluid to disperse.

~ Potato Under Eye Treatment ~

- 1/4 cup of potato
- 1 teaspoon sea salt
- 2 tablespoons of plain yogurt

Finely grate the raw potato then add the remaining ingredients and mix together thoroughly. Chill for at least one hour.

Pat mixture evenly on the face paying particular attention to the under eye area for 10 to 15 minutes then rinse well with warm water.

* SKINSATIONAL TIP:

Potatoes contain an enzyme that helps to diminish dark under eye circles. Reduce swollen under eye bags at the same time by freezing two slices of potato and applying them to the under eye area for up to five minutes.

~ Eye Rescue Balm ~

- 1/4 cup extra virgin olive oil
- 2 tablespoons nettle leaf
- 1 tablespoon parsley

Combine all ingredients together into a mini food processor and process until thoroughly combined. Let mixture infuse together overnight. Strain into a clean container.

Dab around the eye area daily.

* * *

~ *It's the Icing on the Face* ~

- 4 green tea bags
- 1 cup skim milk
- 1 orange
- 2 teaspoons rosemary
- 1 tablespoon organic honey

Brew a strong cup of tea in the skim milk using all the tea bags. Squeeze out the remaining tea from each of the tea bags back into the milk. Finely mince the rosemary and add to the tea. Stir in the freshly squeezed juice from the orange and then add the honey.

Pour mixture into a small ice cube tray and freeze.

Once frozen wrap two of the ice cubes in a face cloth and apply to the under eye area for five minutes. Take the ice cubes off after five minutes to allow the skin to warm then reapply for another five minutes.

* SKINSATIONAL TIP:

The general rule of thumb for swelling is to ice for five minutes on and five minutes off.

~ For Your Eyes Only ~

- 1 tablespoon comfrey
- 2 tablespoons macadamia nut oil
- 1 tablespoon mango
- 2 large cucumber slices

Place the comfrey, nut oil and mango in a mini-food processor and pulse until smooth. Put the mixture into the freezer for 10 to 20 minutes to get cold. Spread a thin layer of the mixture onto each cucumber slice.

Place on under eye area for 15 minutes. Rinse well with warm water.

* * *

~ Eye Spy ~

- 2 chamomile tea bags
- 1/2 cup vitamin water
- 1 tablespoon tomato juice
- 1 tablespoon fresh aloe gel

Microwave vitamin water and tea bags together until bubbling. Squeeze the juice from a small, fresh tomato then express the gel from one large aloe leaf. Mix all ingredients together then let steep until cool.

Squeeze all excess moisture from the tea bags back into the mixture. Place the tea bags in the freezer for 10 to 20 minutes until quite cold.

Position the chilled tea bags on under eye area for 10 minutes. Rinse well with warm water.

Freeze remaining liquid in ice cube trays to use as an under eye cold compress.

* SKINSATIONAL TIP:

Tea is a natural source of tannin which works to help effectively reduce under eye swelling.

~ *Special Occasion* ~
Skin Care Recipe Collection

Just for fun natural skin care recipes! Relax and indulge yourself, your beloved, or friends in a special rejuvenating facial treat.

Have you ever hosted a facial spa party or planned a wonderful romantic facial by firelight with the love of your life? Use these recipes to become inspired and let your creative juices start flowing.

- ❀ Plan a romantic facial treat by stocking up on champagne, getting a fire roaring in the fireplace and lighting the scented candles while you whip up a little magic with a special natural skin care recipe.
- ❀ Host a *Facial Fiesta Party*! Get the whole gang together, rev-up the chocolate fountain and start slathering away. Dipping, sipping, and chocolate facial massage are required. Facial rejuvenation doesn't get much better than that. Yum!
- ❀ Make up a batch of your favorite skin care recipe such as the Love Scrub, package it in a beautifully labeled container and give it as a special gift from the heart.

~ Witches Brew ~

- Carefully select 10 of your best dragon tears, (fresh cranberries can be substituted if necessary)
- Extract 1/4 cup of distilled Viper Venom, (extra virgin olive oil can be used in a pinch)
- Place your smallest cauldron over a very low flame and simmer together slowly until the dragon tears have decomposed in the venom
- Meanwhile in a small skull add one large eye of newt, (an egg yolk will do)
- 2 tablespoons of coarsely chopped Ogre whiskers, (some facial brews occasionally feature fresh rosemary leaves instead)
- Whisk together with 1 tablespoon of gravestone dust, (in the case of allergic reactions kosher or sea salt are alternatives)
- Strain the contents of the cauldron very slowly into the skull while chanting and whisking vigorously to thicken into a smooth, rich potion.

Apply the bewitched potion liberally with a gryphon feather, (or small facial brush), and allow to set for 15 to 20 minutes.

Rinse completely with warmed goblin guts ~ strained of course, (though water will work just as well).

Just Boootiful!

* * *

~ *Passion Peel* ~

- 1 egg white
- 1/2 passion fruit
- 1 tablespoon cornstarch
- 2 tablespoons clover honey

Whip egg whites until stiff. Slowly sprinkle in the cornstarch while continuing to whip until thoroughly combined. Mash the passion fruit into a soft smooth pulp stirring in the honey.

Fold the passion fruit mixture into the egg whites until thoroughly incorporated.

Apply peel and let set for 20 minutes. Rinse well with warm water.

* * *

~ *May Day Moisturizer* ~

- 1/4 cup sunflower oil
- 1/4 cup grapefruit juice

- 1 tablespoon fresh aloe vera gel
- 3 to 4 fresh peppermint leaves

Finely chop the peppermint leaves. Combine all ingredients together in a small bottle. Cover and shake well. Let ingredients infuse together overnight. Strain out the peppermint leaves if desired.

Gently massage a small amount of the moisturizer into skin.

* * *

~ *Flower Power Scrub* ~

- 2 sprigs lavender
- 1 tablespoon safflower oil
- 2 tablespoons epsom salts
- 1/8 cup blue violets
- 1 rose bud

Combine all ingredients in a food processor and blend until thoroughly pureed.

Use to gently scrub face. Rinse well with warm water.

* * *

~ *Valentine Rose Spritz* ~

- 1/2 cup rose petals
- 1/4 cup rose hips
- 2 tablespoons chamomile tea leaves

- 1 tablespoon castor oil
- 1 cup spring water

Roughly chop both rose petals and rose hips. Combine all ingredients in a small saucepan and simmer over medium low heat for 20 minutes. Let cool completely before straining into a misting bottle.

Spritz skin as desired throughout the day.

* * *

~ *Magical Holiday Eggnog Mask* ~

- 1 egg yolk
- 1/4 cup heavy cream
- 1/4 teaspoon vanilla bean
- 1/4 cup soy flour

With the tip of a small knife gently remove the pulp from the inside of the vanilla bean. Whisk all ingredients together until frothy.

Apply mask for up to 20 minutes. Rinse well with warm water.

* * *

~ *Sparkling Irish Eyes* ~

- 2/3 cups heavy cream

- 2 teaspoons fresh sage
- 1 medium potato

Finely chop the sage then grate the potato. Combine all ingredients into a small saucepan and simmer together over low heat until the potato is cooked and the liquid is reduced by half.

Cool mixture in the freezer until quite cold then form two small patties.

Apply one under each eye for 10 minutes. Rinse well with warm water.

* * *

~ New Years Facial Celebration ~

- 1 teaspoon honey
- 1/2 cup cantaloupe
- 3 tablespoons cornstarch
- 1/4 cup champagne vinegar

Roughly chop the cantaloupe then add all ingredients into a blender. Whip together until smooth.

Apply mask for up to 20 minutes. Rinse well with warm water.

* SKINSATIONAL TIP:

Castor oil is especially rich in moisturizing properties and an ideal choice for sensitive and dry skin types.

~ Spring Fling Spritz ~

- 1 1/2 cups mineral water
- 1/4 cup strawberries
- 1/2 cup strawberry leaves
- 1 tablespoon castor oil
- 1 sprig rosemary and thyme
- 1 lemon

Roughly chop the strawberries, strawberry leaves, rosemary, thyme and lemon. Combine all ingredients in a small saucepan and simmer over medium low heat until strawberries begin to fall apart.

Press mixture through a sieve while straining into a small spray mist bottle. Spritz skin throughout the day as needed.

* * *

~ Acne Independence Face Scrub ~

- 1/4 cup cornmeal
- 8 plain aspirin
- 1 tablespoon baking soda

- 2 small birch leaves
- 1/3 cup cider vinegar

Puree all ingredients together in a food processor until smooth. Let mixture infuse overnight then strain into a clean container.

Use as a facial scrub once daily. Rinse well with lukewarm water.

---

* SKINSATIONAL TIP:

Spot treat blemishes by lightly moistening a plain, uncoated aspirin tablet and rubbing it on the emerging blemish or make a thin paste by dissolving the aspirin tablet in a tiny drop of water. The salicylic acid in the aspirin makes an excellent and effective spot treatment.

~ Ghostly Vapors ~

- 2 cups distilled water
- 1/4 cup dry instant milk powder
- 1/4 cup loosely packed peppermint leaves
- 2 tablespoons almond oil

Combine all ingredients in saucepan. Bring to a boil and remove from heat.

Cool slightly before using as a facial steam.

~ *Pumpkin Patch* ~

- 1/2 cup cider vinegar
- 5 to 6 thin slices of pumpkin
- 1 teaspoon sage
- 2 tablespoon raw sugar

Add the pumpkin slices to a small saucepan. Combine the remaining ingredients and simmer over medium low heat until pumpkin is softened slightly.

Drain the pumpkin slices on paper towell until slightly cooled.

Arrange pumpkin slices carefully on the face, covering the under eye area, cheeks, forehead and chin.

Leave on for up to 15 minutes. Rinse well with warm water.

* * *

~ *Love Scrub* ~

- 1/2 pomegranate
- 2 tablespoons raw sugar
- 1 tablespoon almond oil
- 1 tablespoon honey

Scoop out pomegranate into mini-food processor. Add remaining ingredients and process mixture until smooth.

Use to scrub face gently. Rinse well with warm water.

* SKINSATIONAL TIP:

The pomegranate tree has been said to originate in the Garden of Eden and been used extensively since early Egyptian times for its medicinal properties.

~ The Monster Mash ~

- 1/2 avocado
- 1 lemon
- 2 tablespoon sea salt or kosher salt
- 1 to 2 teaspoons of honey

Mash the avocado until smooth. Mix in the freshly squeezed juice of the lemon. Add the remaining ingredients and continue to mash the mixture into the consistency of a thick paste.

Gently use to scrub your face. Rinse well with warm water.

* * *

~ Easter Egg Wash ~

- 3 tablespoons lime juice
- 1 egg
- 1/8 cup corn meal

Whip egg until frothy. Fold in freshly squeezed lime juice then slowly stir in the cornmeal.

Use to cleanse skin. Rinse well with warm water.

. . . .

* SKINSATIONAL TIP:

Saturate the end of a Q-tip in freshly squeezed citrus juice such as orange, lemon or lime and dab on age spots or freckles as a natural skin lightening treatment.

. . . .

~ *Moisturizing Mardi Gras* ~

- 1/2 cup walnut oil
- 1/4 cup blue violet blossoms
- 1/4 cup pansy petals
- 1 tablespoon chopped lemon balm
- 1 teaspoon epsom salts

Roughly chop the violets, pansies, and lemon balm. Combine all ingredients in a small container and let infuse together for several hours or overnight.

Strain into a clean container and use to moisturize skin daily.

~ *Boo Berry Balm* ~

- 1/4 cup raspberries
- 1/8 cup blueberries
- 1/4 cup coconut milk
- 2 tablespoons cornstarch
- 1 teaspoon castor oil

Gently heat all ingredients in a small saucepan on medium low until berries are soft and mushy. Transfer to a food processor and pulse until smooth. Let mixture cool slightly.

Apply for 15 minutes. Rinse well with warm water.

***

* SKINSATIONAL TIP:

The USDA identifies wild blueberries as rich in anthocyanins which gives the skin of the fruit such a deep color as well as one of the highest in antioxidant activity. Red cherries and purple grapes are other sources and considered to be an asset in anti-aging routines.

***

~ *Spooktacular Peel* ~

- In your smallest skull slowly simmer 1/8 cup blue goblin eyeballs (blueberries), 1/8 cup harden vampire

bat blood (cranberries), and 1/8 cup viper venom (apple cider vinegar) until the moon rises over the horizon and the ingredients have all decomposed
- Use a cobweb (sieve) to mash and strain the brew into your favorite cauldron, add one packet of dried and crushed ogre bones (plain gelatin)
- Meanwhile, briskly whisk the whites of one separated dragon egg (egg white) until stiff
- Fold all ingredients together

Apply to wart infested skin for up to 20 minutes with a phoenix feather.

Rinse well with warm monster tears, (or water of course).

---

* SKINSATIONAL TIP:

Jojoba oil is readily absorbed by the skin and has a range of anti-aging properties when used as a moisturizing oil. It is a natural antibacterial and antioxidant that works to promote healing and to restore skin elasticity.

~ Birthday Bee Balm ~

- 5 bee balm blossoms
- 1/4 cup shea butter
- 2 tablespoons aloe vera

Express gel from a large aloe leaf and combine with remaining ingredients into a blender. Blend on high until completely combined.

Apply for up to 25 minutes. Rinse well with warm water.

~ Natural Skin Care Ingredients and Their Properties ~

The properties of natural skin care ingredients describe the attributes and qualities that each natural ingredient contributes to the topical treatment of aging skin conditions.

The properties of natural ingredients that are beneficial for the skin and contribute to skin rejuvenation include the following attributes:

Antibacterial	Antibiotic
Antifungal	Anti-inflammatory
Antimicrobial	Antioxidant
Antiseptic	Astringent
Cell Repair	Cell Regeneration
Cleansing	Demulcent
Detoxification	Disinfectant
Emollient	Exfoliation
Firming	Healing
Humectant	Hydration
Lightening	Moisturizing
Softening Agent	Stimulant

When preparing skin care recipes it is important to understand that each ingredient will contribute its own distinctive properties to the recipes which are formulated to provide essential nourishment to aging skin in order to stimulate facial rejuvenation.

~ A ~

Almond- Used in scrubs to exfoliate skin. Attributes include moisturizing and emollient properties. Particularly rich in vitamin A.

Almond Oil- Moisturizing, skin softening and emollient qualities which can be readily absorbed by the skin. Especially beneficial for dry and sensitive skin types.

Aloe Vera- Healing, anti-inflammatory, cleansing, and moisturizing properties. Also works to strengthen skin tissue, acts as a skin softener, and to improve skin elasticity.

Apple- A malic acid that serves to gently exfoliate and cleanse.

Apple Cider Vinegar- Primary property is malic acid which aids in the exfoliation of dead skin cells, has astringent and anti-bacterial properties.

Apricots- Antioxidant, demulcent and soothing properties. Excellent treatment for dry, sensitive and scaly skin.

Arrowroot- Astringent properties, ideal for acne prone skin.

Aspirin- A beta hydroxyl acid, (salicylic acid), used as an exfoliant with anti-inflammatory properties. Excellent option for oily, acne prone skin.

Avocado- Rich in vitamin E, an emollient as well as a moisturizer.

~ B ~

Baking Soda- Mild exfoliant and cleanser with astringent properties. Excellent for acne prone skin.

Banana- Rich in vitamins A and C, moisturizing and emollient qualities.

Barley- An antibacterial and emollient that helps to refine pores and retard wrinkles.

Bee Balm- Antiseptic, anti-inflammatory, healing as well as skin soothing properties.

Beet- Rich in folic acid which helps to stimulate cell renewal as well as moisturizes the skin.

Birch Leaves- Used medicinally as a disinfectant, antiseptic and to reduce skin inflammations. Also an astringent which makes it perfect for oily and acne prone skin.

Blackberries- Antioxidant, astringent, rich in vitamins C and E.

Black Tea- Stimulates skin cells, anti-inflammatory, antioxidant and antibacterial properties.

Blueberries- Antioxidant rich in vitamins, helps to protect and repair the skin.

Bran- An emollient, reduces pore size.

Buttermilk- A lactic acid which has moisturizing, exfoliant and cleansing properties.

~ C ~

Calendula- A humectant with astringent, antiseptic, antimicrobial, healing, anti-inflammatory properties as well as a natural source of salicylic acid.

Carrot- Rich in high levels of beta carotene, exfoliant with moisturizing properties.

Castor Oil- A rich moisturizer, soothes itchy skin. Great treatment for around the sensitive eye area and for dry skin types.

Chamomile- Tones, has healing and anti-inflammatory properties.

Cherries- Antioxidant, anti-inflammatory, rich in vitamins C and E.

Cocoa Butter- A rich moisturizer and emollient. Especially beneficial for dry and sensitive skin types.

Coconut Oil- Healing properties, antibacterial, antifungal, antimicrobial, antioxidant, easily absorbed by the skin.

Comfrey- Healing, astringent, emollient, anti-inflammatory, stimulates cell renewal as well as used as an effective scar and acne treatment.

Cornflower- An antioxidant that is also used for its astringent, and antibacterial properties as well as soothing inflamed and irritated skin.

Cornmeal- An emollient that helps to refine pores.

Corn Oil- Moisturizer, emollient.

Cornstarch- Softens skin as well as used as an absorbent and a thickening agent in natural skin care recipes.

Corn Syrup- An emollient that also has humectant properties.

Cranberries- Antioxidant, antibacterial, rich in vitamin C.

Cream- A lactic acid, gentle exfoliant, cleanser.

Cream of Tartar- Cleansing properties, softens skin.

Cucumber- Antioxidant properties, soothing, can be used to reduce under eye puffiness and wrinkles.

~ D ~

Dandelion- Astringent, antibacterial, and healing properties; helps reduce acne and prevent outbreaks.

~ E ~

Echinacea- A skin rejuvenation favorite due to properties that include the ability to strengthen skin tissue which serve to firm sagginess as well as for the healing properties, promotion of cell regeneration, natural antibiotic, and reduction of skin inflammation.

Egg- An emollient; the whites condition the skin leaving it soft and silky. Typically used in facial mask and skin peel recipes to tighten the skin. Egg whites are usually used for oily skin types while the yolks are used for sensitive and dry skin types. Egg yolks are rich in vitamins A, D and E.

Elderberry Flowers- Mild astringent, hydrates dry skin, anti-inflammatory, skin softener, cleanses, and stimulant properties.

Epsom Salts- Dries out oily skin and reduces acne outbreaks.

Evening Primrose- Antioxidant, anti-inflammatory, heals and protects.

Eyebright- Astringent, and antibiotic properties as well as reduces inflammation and swelling.

~ F ~

Fennel- Antiseptic, anti-inflammatory, helps prevent wrinkles.

Flax Seed Oil- An emollient that also prevents scarring and helps treat stretch marks.

Fuchsia- Calms irritated skin, soothing, mild emollient.

~ G ~

Garlic- Natural antibiotic, antiseptic, antibacterial.

Gelatin- Skin softener, helps to tighten sagging skin, used as a binder.

Geranium- Astringent, antiseptic and healing properties.

Ginger- Anti-inflammatory, stimulates circulation.

Grapefruit- Antioxidant, exfoliating properties, one of the more powerful fruit acids for treating aging skin concerns.

Grapes- Antioxidant, promotes healing, anti-inflammatory, protects the skin from damage, and improves skin elasticity.

Green Tea- Antioxidant, antibacterial, anti-inflammatory, rich in vitamins B, C, and E.

~ H~

Hazelnut Oil- Emollient and moisturizing properties. Especially beneficial for dry, sensitive skin types.

Hibiscus- Antioxidant, astringent, and anti-inflammatory properties, also improves skin elasticity and moisture content.

Hollyhock- Moisturizing and emollient properties.

Honey- Antibacterial, antimicrobial and healing properties. It is also an excellent moisturizer and skin softener; helps prevent wrinkles as well as acne outbreaks.

~ J ~

Jasmine- Anti-inflammatory, astringent, and antibacterial.

Jojoba Oil- Antibacterial, antioxidant, and healing properties as well as a moisturizer and skin softener, can help restore elasticity. Particularly noted to absorb into the skin with ease. An excellent ingredient in anti-aging skin care recipes to address wrinkles as well as acne prone skin.

Juniper Berries- Natural antibiotic, antiseptic, antibacterial, and astringent.

~ K ~

Kiwi- Antioxidant, rich in vitamin C and E.

~ L ~

Lard- A skin softening agent, an emollient and moisturizer.

Lavender- Antiseptic, antibacterial, stimulant, healing, promotes cell activity and regeneration.

Lemon Balm- Antibiotic and healing properties.

Lemongrass- Cleanses, reduces inflammation, calms irritated skin, has antioxidant properties as well as antiseptic, astringent, antibacterial, and antifungal properties. A particularly good choice for acne prone skin.

Lettuce- Emollient and analgesic properties as well as a skin conditioner.

Licorice- Healing, anti-inflammatory, emollient, cleansing, and skin lightening properties.

Lime- An alpha hydroxyl acid, exfoliant properties, one of the more powerful of the fruit acids. Highly recommended for anti-aging skin care regimens.

~ M ~

Macadamia Nut Oil- Emollient, moisturizer, easily absorbed by the skin.

Malva- Healing, anti-inflammatory, emollient, skin softener as well as a natural acne remedy. Rich in vitamins A, B, C, and E.

Mango- Healing, emollient, skin softener, astringent, and skin stimulant. Rich in vitamin C.

Marigold- Astringent, cleansing, healing, and cell regeneration properties. An excellent natural skin care ingredient for acne prone skin.

Marjoram- Healing, anti-inflammatory, antiseptic, and antibacterial. A good choice for oily and acne prone skin.

Mayonnaise- A lactic acid which helps to cleanse the skin with the emollient qualities of eggs.

Milk- A lactic acid which gently cleanses and exfoliates.

Mineral Oil- Moisturizer, emollient properties

Mint- Stimulates skin cells, astringent and antiseptic properties.

~ N ~

Nasturtium- Healing, antibacterial, anti-inflammatory, and antibiotic properties. Also rich in vitamin C.

Nectarine- Antioxidant, rich in vitamin A.

Nettle- A natural cleanser, an emollient and also used to calm irritated skin. A particularly good choice for dry and sensitive skin types.

~ O ~

Oatmeal- An emollient, skin softener, calms irritated skin, and relieves itching.

Olive Leaf- An antiseptic, antibacterial, with healing properties.

Olive Oil- Rich emollient, anti-inflammatory, and antioxidant qualities.

Orange- An alpha hydroxyl acid which gently exfoliates, and also has antiseptic properties. Rich in vitamins A, B, and C.

Oregano- Healing and antiseptic properties as well as an antioxidant.

~ P ~

Pansy- An emollient that cleanses and also has healing properties in addition to calming skin irritations.

Papaya- Rich in papain which is used in meat tenderizing formulas. Serves as an effective skin softener, mild exfoliant with gentle bleaching properties.

Parsley- Healing and anti-inflammatory properties.

Passion Fruit- Antioxidant, exfoliant, and antibacterial properties. Considered as one of the most powerful of fruit acids. An excellent ingredient for natural anti-aging skin care recipes.

PawPaw- Antioxidant and healing properties. Noted for treating acne.

Peaches- Antioxidant and emollient properties. Rich in vitamin C and carotene. Especially beneficial for dry or sensitive skin types.

Peanut Oil- Emollient and moisturizing properties.

Peppermint- Anti-inflammatory, cleansing, and antibacterial properties while soothing irritated skin in addition to stimulating skin cells, restoring elasticity, tones, tightens pores, reduces swelling, reduces redness and a variety of other skin irritations. It is good choice for oily and acne prone skin.

Pineapple- Antioxidant properties as well as a mild cleanser. Helps to tone skin and used as an exfoliant.

Plum- Antioxidant with mild astringent properties.

Pomegranate- One of the more powerful antioxidants, as well as a strong astringent.

Potato- Emollient, anti-inflammatory, and skin softening properties. Helps to reduce dark under eye circles and under eye puffiness.

Powdered Milk- Gentle cleanser and exfoliant.

Pumpkin- Exfoliant, skin softening properties.

~ R ~

Raspberries- Antioxidant, astringent, antibacterial and antimicrobial properties.

Red Clover- A strong antioxidant with healing and skin softening properties. Used to treat a variety of chronic skin irritations.

Rhubarb- Antioxidant, cleansing, and astringent properties.

Rose Hips and Petals- Rich source of vitamin C which helps stimulates collagen production as well as has healing, astringent, emollient and skin softening properties. A popular ingredient used by cosmetic companies in anti-aging skin care treatments to fight wrinkles, fine lines, combat the effects of sun damaged skin, promotes tissue regeneration as well as to reduce scars. Hydrates and protects the skin as well.

Rosemary- Astringent, stimulates circulation, antibacterial and restores elasticity to the skin. An ideal choice for aging skin, acne prevention as well as for oily skin types.

~ S ~

Safflower Oil- Emollient and moisturizing properties. Rich in fatty acids which promotes cell regeneration. Easily absorbed by the skin. An excellent oil for aging, dry and sensitive skin types.

Sage- An antioxidant, antiseptic and antibacterial as well as used as a cleanser, and to tone skin. Properties also include the ability to increase circulation, reduce pore size and restore elasticity. A good choice for both oily and aging skin.

Salt- Exfoliates and stimulates the skin.

Sea Buckthorn- Healing, moisturizing and cell regeneration properties. Rich in vitamins A and E.

Seaweed- Rich in nutrients, vitamins especially B12, A, C, E, K, folic acid, niacin and pantothenic acid and minerals- calcium, potassium, iron, zinc, sodium, and magnesium- that are absorbed by the skin. Properties include cleansing, toning, hydrating, stimulating cell regeneration, and healing.

Sesame Oil- Emollient, moisturizing, and antibacterial properties. Rich in vitamin E.

Shea Butter- Emollient, healing, anti-inflammatory, skin softening, moisturizing and antioxidant properties as well as provides natural UV protection from the sun.

Sour Cream- Mild cleanser with the gentle exfoliant properties of a lactic acid.

Soy- Healing, antioxidant, moisturizing, and skin softening properties. Promotes cell regeneration and restores elasticity. Rich in vitamin E. An excellent natural anti-aging skin care ingredient.

Spearmint- Antiseptic, astringent and skin stimulant.

St. John's Wort- Soothing, anti-inflammatory, and antibacterial attributes.

Strawberry- Antioxidant which helps protect and repair the skin. Tones and helps to control acne outbreaks.

Sunflower Oil- Regenerates, emollient, moisturizes, rich in vitamins A and E. An excellent oil for treating aging skin concerns.

Sweet Potato- Antioxidant, anti-inflammatory, and healing properties. Rich in vitamin A (in the form of beta-carotene) and vitamin C.

~ T ~

Tapioca- A demulcent as well as a gentle exfoliant. Helps to tighten skin and to sooth inflamed skin.

Thyme- Has astringent properties, antiseptic, natural antibiotic, and anti-fungal properties as well as aids in healing, has skin protective properties, reduces inflammation, and stimulates the skin. An especially good herb to use for acne prone and aging skin.

Tomato- Antioxidant, exfoliant, and rich in lycopene (the highest levels of which are found in the skin) as well as vitamins C and A.

Turnip- Reduces blotchiness and skin redness.

~ V ~

Vinegar- Exfoliant, antibacterial, anti-inflammatory, cleansing, skin softening, detoxifies as well as possesses strong astringent properties. Natural vinegars such as apple cider, white wine, balsamic, rice, coconut, and fruit fermented vinegars are effective choices in anti-aging skin care recipes lending the benefits of tartaric and citric acid as well as a wide range of rejuvenating properties.

Violets- Antibacterial, emollient, skin softener, and healing properties as well as detoxifies the skin. Beneficial for aging, acne prone, and dry skin types.

~ W ~

Walnut Oil- Moisturizer, emollient

Wheat Germ- Used as a mild exfoliant with moisturizing properties.

Wheat Germ Oil- Emollient and moisturizer as well as helps to refine pores.

Witch Hazel- Astringent, anti-inflammatory, and healing properties as well as an excellent oil absorbing skin toner to tighten skin tissue, reduce broken capillaries and treat bruises. A wonderful, all purpose herb for facial rejuvenation recipes. The leaves and bark are the parts of the plant used in skin care recipes.

~ Y ~

Yarrow- Astringent, cleanses and tones. Helps to tighten skin, reduce pore size and prevent acne outbreaks along with soothing the skin. Especially beneficial for oily, and acne prone skin as well as aging skin concerns.

Yeast- Antibacterial properties and helps restore ph balance to the skin.

Yogurt- A lactic acid (an AHA, alpha hydroxyl acid) which is a gentle exfoliator especially for sensitive skin types. Also has emollient properties.

~ Resources ~

Anti-Aging Skin Care and
Facial Rejuvenation Information

---

http://www.skincareresourcecenter.com

(Of course!) ☺

Online Natural Skin Care and Facial
Rejuvenation Product Resources:
For selection, quality and price
our favorite picks are:

---

http://www.skincareresourcecenter.com/best-skin-care-product-resources.html

---

Natural Skin Care Recipe Card Sampler

---

http://www.skincareresourcecenter.com/natural-skin-care-recipes.html

~ References ~

- A Consumer's Dictionary of Cosmetic Ingredients: Complete Information About the Harmful and Desirable Ingredients Found in Cosmetics and Cosmeceuticals by Ruth Winter
- Encyclopedia of Common Natural Ingredients: Used in Food, Drugs, and Cosmetics by Albert Y. Leung and Steven Foster
- Foods and Nutrition Encyclopedia by Ensminger AH, Ensminger, ME, Kondale JE, Robson JRK: Pegus Press, Clovis, California 1983
- Food for Health: A Nutrition Encyclopedia by Ensminger AH, Esminger M. K. J. e. al: Pegus Press, Clovis, California, 1986
- Skin Care and Cosmetic Ingredients Dictionary-(Milady's Skin Care and Cosmetics Ingredients Dictionary) by Natalia Michalun and Varinia Michalun
- The Complete Woman's Herbal by Anne McIntyre: Henry Holt & Co., NY 1995
- The Complete Medicinal Herbal by Penelope Ody: Dorling Kindersley Ltd, London 1993
- The Herbal Body Book by Jeanne Rose: Grosset & Dunlap, NY 1976

- <u>The Visual Foods Encyclopedia,</u> Fortin, Francois, Editorial Director: Macmillan, New York 1996
- <u>The Whole Foods Encyclopedia</u> by Rebecca Wood: Prentice-Hall Press, New York, NY 1988

~ *Internet Reference Sources* ~

- Botanical.com
- Botanical-online.com
- Britannica.com
- CosmeticCop.com
- DermaDoctor.com
- Dermsmart.com- Skin Encyclopedia
- Encyclopedia.com
- FDA.gov
- Health-Cares.net
- Internethealthlibrary.com
- Merck.com
- Resources.ciheam.org
- Skincaredictionary.com
- Wikipedia.org